Emerging and Re-emerging Infectious Diseases

Emerging and Re-emerging Infectious Diseases

Editor-in-Chief

Tarun Kumar Dutta
Professor and Head
Department of Medicine
Jawaharlal Institute of Postgraduate Medical Education and Research
Puducherry, India

Editors

Subhash Chandra Parija
Professor and Head
Department of Microbiology
Jawaharlal Institute of Postgraduate Medical Education and Research
Puducherry, India

Jamini Kanta Dutta
Consultant Physician
Formerly Medical Superintendent-cum-Consultant
Infectious Diseases Hospital, Kingsway Camp
Delhi, India

JAYPEE BROTHERS MEDICAL PUBLISHERS (P) LTD

New Delhi • Panama City • London • Dhaka • Kathmandu

Jaypee Brothers Medical Publishers (P) Ltd

Headquarter

Jaypee Brothers Medical Publishers (P) Ltd
4838/24, Ansari Road, Daryaganj
New Delhi 110 002, India
Phone: +91-11-43574357
Fax: +91-11-43574314
Email: jaypee@jaypeebrothers.com

Overseas Offices

J.P. Medical Ltd.,
83 Victoria Street, London
SW1H 0HW (UK)
Phone: +44-2031708910
Fax: +02-03-0086180
Email: info@jpmedpub.com

Jaypee-Highlights Medical Publishers Inc.
City of Knowledge, Bld. 237, Clayton
Panama City, Panama
Phone: +507-301-0496
Fax: +507-301-0499
Email: cservice@jphmedical.com

Jaypee Brothers Medical Publishers (P) Ltd
17/1-B Babar Road, Block-B
Shaymali, Mohammadpur
Dhaka-1207, Bangladesh
Mobile: +08801912003485
Email: jaypeedhaka@gmail.com

Jaypee Brothers Medical Publishers (P) Ltd
Shorakhute
Kathmandu, Nepal
Phone: +00977-9841528578
Email: jaypee.nepal@gmail.com

Website: www.jaypeebrothers.com
Website: www.jaypeedigital.com

Inquiries for bulk sales may be solicited at: jaypee@jaypeebrothers.com

Emerging and Re-emerging Infectious Diseases

First Edition: **2012,** Reprint: 2027

ISBN: 978-93-5025-960-3

Printed in India

Dedicated to

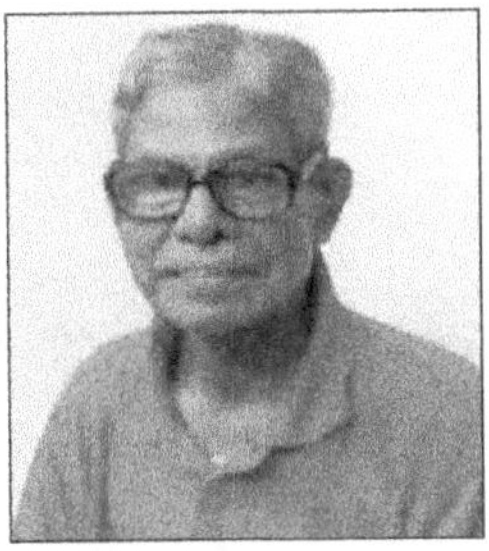

28 April 1924 – 17 October 2007

Memory of my father late JK Dutta who was Medical Superintendent of Infectious Diseases Hospital, Kingsway Camp, Delhi, India and had inspired me into the field of tropical diseases.

TK Dutta

Contributors

Amitabh Giri
Sonologist
Sonoscan and Zenith CT Scan (P) Ltd
Balasore, Odisha, India

D Kumar
Department of Parasitology
Rajiv Gandhi College of Veterinary and Animal Sciences
Kurumbapet, Puducherry, India

DM Thappa
Professor and Head
Department of Dermatology and Sexually Transmitted Disease
Jawaharlal Institute of Postgraduate Medical Education and Research
Puducherry, India

Late BK Giri
Consultant Physician and Pediatrician
Sonoscan, Balasore, Odisha, India

Late JK Dutta
Former Medical Superintendent cum consultant
Infectious Diseases Hospital
Kingsway Camp, Delhi, India

LK Das
Scientist E
Vector Control Research Center
(Indian Council of Medical Research)
Indira Nagar, Puducherry, India

Madhumala Giri
Consultant physician and Gastrointestinal Endoscopist
Sonoscan, Balasore, Odisha, India

PS Sahu
Department of Microbiology
Alluri Sitarama Raju Academy of Medical Sciences
West Godavari District
Eluru, Andhra Pradesh, India

RK Sahoo
Professor
Department of Medicine
Postgraduate Institute of Medical Education and Research
Ram Manohar Lohia Hospital
New Delhi, India

SC Parija
Professor and Head
Department of Microbiology
Jawaharlal Institute of Postgraduate Medical Education and Research
Puducherry, India

SP Pani
Ex Deputy Director (Senior Grade)
Vector Control Research Center
(Indian Council of Medical Research)
Indira Nagar, Puducherry, India

T Talukdar
Associate Professor
Tuberculosis and Chest Diseases
Lady Hardinge Medical College
New Delhi, India

TK Dutta
Professor and Head
Department of Medicine
Jawaharlal Institute of Postgraduate Medical Education and Research
Puducherry, India

V Mukta
Assistant Professor
Department of Medicine
Jawaharlal Institute of Postgraduate Medical Education and Research
Puducherry, India

PREFACE

The book was the brainchild of Dr JK Dutta, former Medical Superintendent of Infectious Diseases Hospital, Kingsway Camp, Delhi, India. He initiated its compilation. However, he did not live long to see the publication of this book. By virtue of his education and training in Tropical Medicine in Edinburgh University, UK, he had developed profound interest in infectious diseases.

Smallpox has been eradicated from the globe. Diseases like diphtheria, whooping cough, poliomyelitis and dracunculosis are on the verge of eradication. However, new diseases have emerged and some old diseases have re-emerged in India and other parts of the globe; to mention a few, they are chikungunya fever, Hanta virus pulmonary syndrome, Lyme disease, West Nile encephalitis, cryptosporidiosis, cyclosporiasis, transmissible spongiform encephalopathy, HIV/AIDS, avian influenza, transfusion and transplant-related diseases. The aim of this book is to highlight selected problems with new and old diseases, e.g. transplantation rabies and rabies transmitted by bats, coinfection of tuberculosis and HIV, etc. The book also emphasizes on recent advances in diagnosis and treatment of various infectious diseases. It has a general section on infectious diseases and their prevention. Authors of various chapters are experienced workers in their field and thus there are plenty of references in this book. The book is expected to be of immense help to physicians, microbiologists, and pediatricians—both budding and established.

Not the least, my sincere thanks to Mr Puneet Mishra for helping to prepare the manuscript of this book.

Any suggestion is welcome.
Reader's satisfaction, Author's success.

TK Dutta

Acknowledgments

I am thankful to Dr BC Roy awardee, Dr SC Parija, Professor and Head, Department of Microbiology of Jawaharlal Institute of Postgraduate Medical Education and Research, Puducherry, India for suggesting the title of this book as "Emerging and Re-emerging Infectious Diseases."

Contents

Section A: General Aspects

Section B: Infectious Diseases

Section C: Appendices

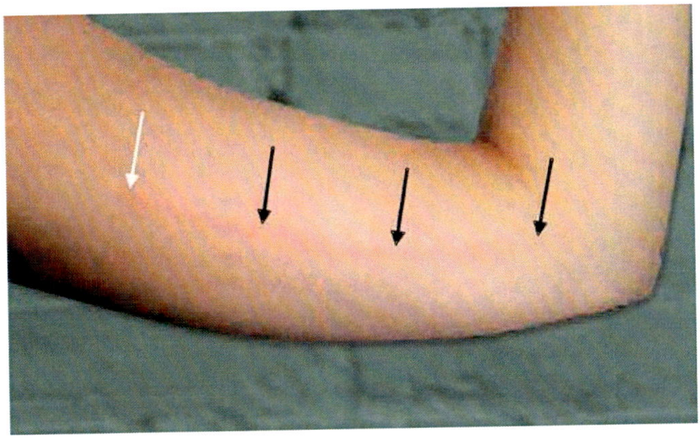

Fig. 28.1: Lymphangitis

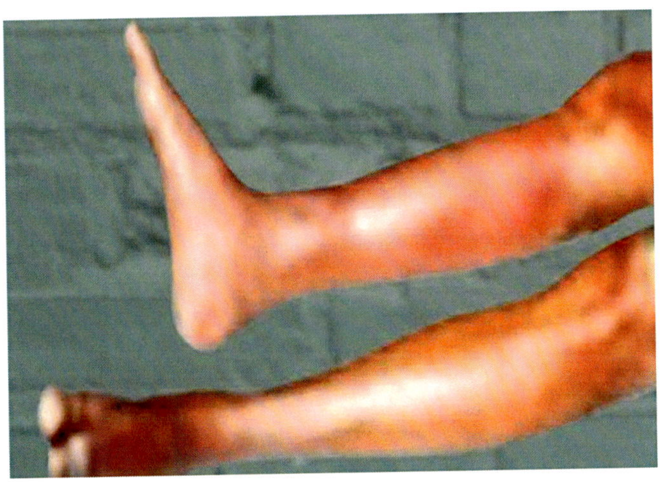

Fig. 28.2: Dermato-lymphangitis of right leg

Plate 2

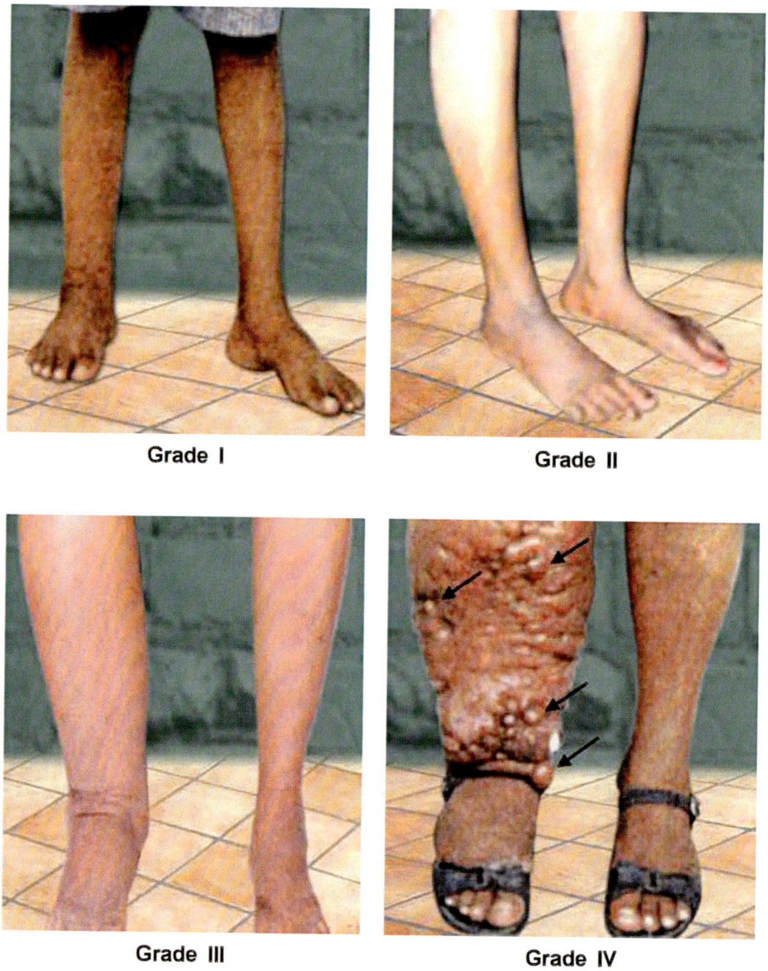

Fig. 28.4: Lymphedema grades of lower extremity

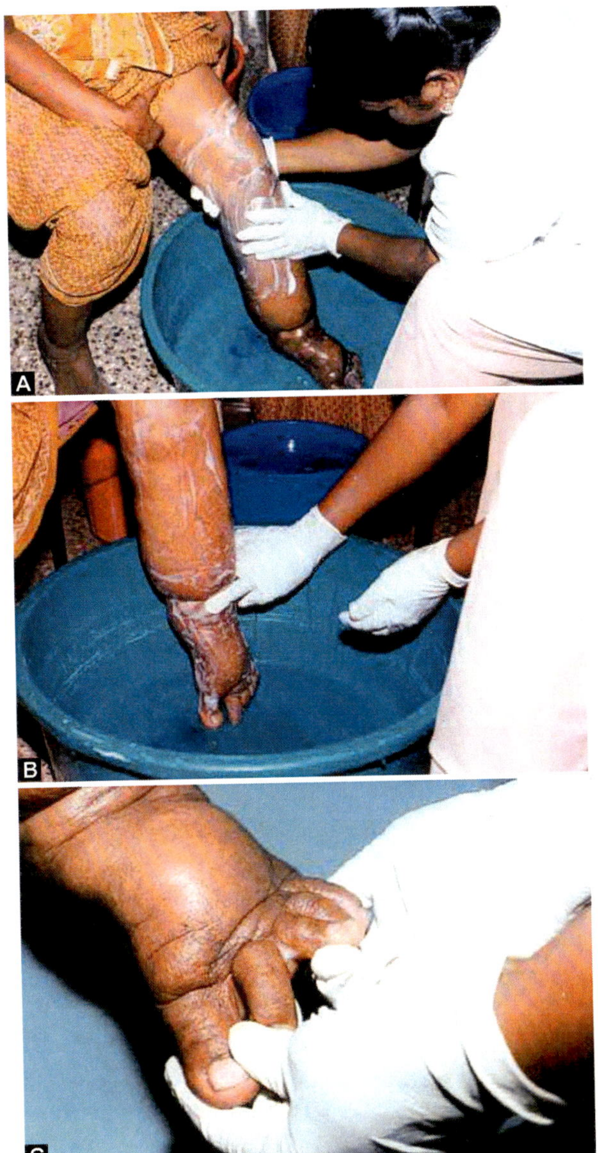

Figs 28.7A to C: (A) Washing soap and water; (B) Cleaning folds
(C) Looking for entry lesions

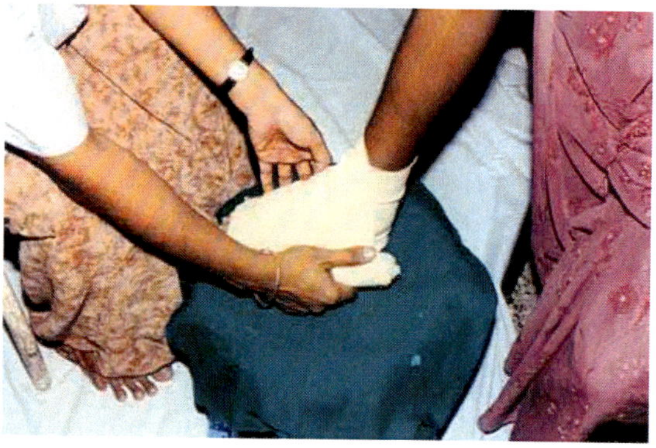

Fig. 28.8(A): Use of pressure bandage

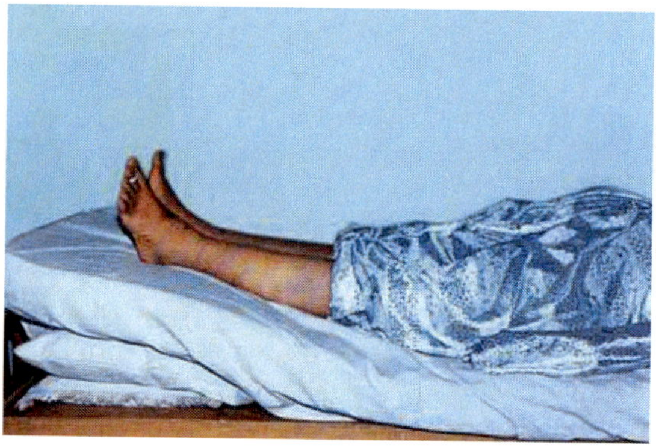

Fig. 28.8(C): Limb elevation

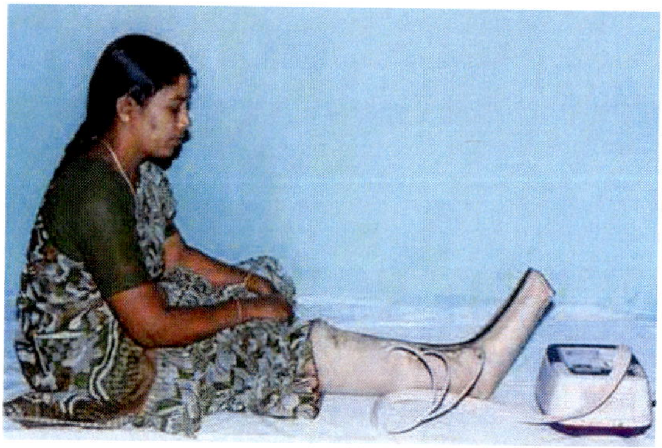

Fig. 28.8(D): Pneumatic compression

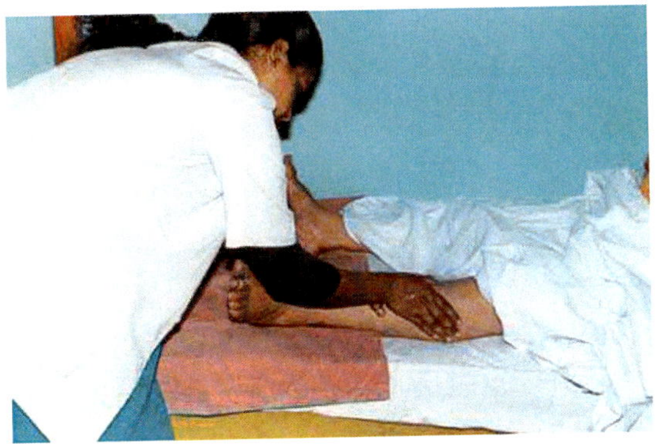

Fig. 28.8(E): Manual massage

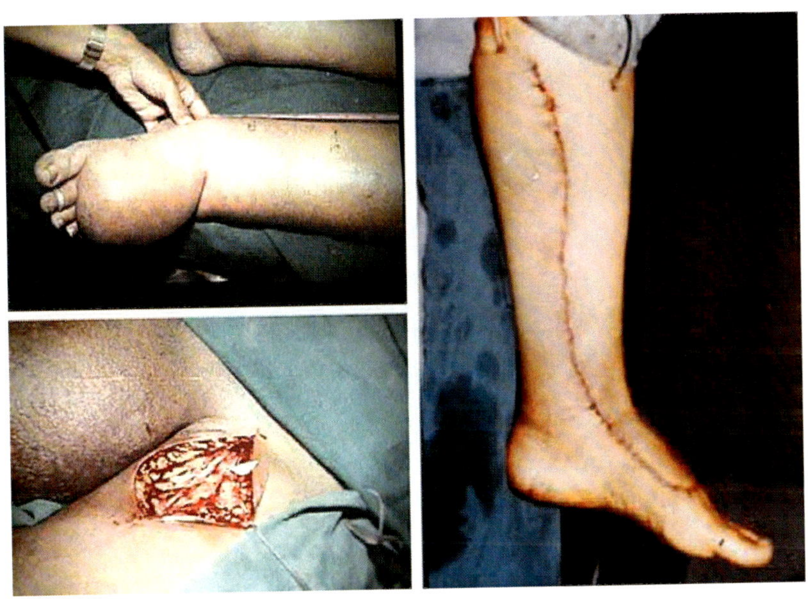

Fig. 28.9: Lymphonodo-venous shunt

Section A

General Aspects

1

Chapter

Prevention of Communicable Diseases: Vaccines Today and Tomorrow

JK Dutta

Prevention of communicable diseases is a prime priority in India. Immunization for prevention of some diseases of childhood is a well established practice. The national immunization program in India is known as Universal Immunization Program (UIP). Immunization against diphtheria, tetanus, pertussis, tuberculosis, polio and measles is carried out under UIP in India at present **(Table 1.1)**.

The schedule of immunization under the program is noted below.

VACCINES MEANT FOR ADULTS

Typhoid Vaccine

Salmonellosis causes typhoid and paratyphoid fever in several countries even now including in India. Protective vaccination is recommended to prevent the infection both among travelers and indigenous population.

Types of Vaccines Available

1. Vi capsular polysaccharide antigen vaccine (VICPS).
2. Acetone inactivated vaccine.
3. Ty21a oral vaccine.

Table 1.1: Universal immunization program schedule (1983)

Vaccines/Toxoid	*Age*
DPT	6,10,14 weeks, 16–18 months
OPV	6,10,14 weeks, 16–18 months
BCG	Birth or 6 weeks
Measles	9 months and above
DT	5 years
TT	10 and 16 years

Pregnant women should receive at least 2 doses of tetanus toxoid at interval of 4 weeks

Primary Vaccination Schedule

a. **VICPS:** VICPS should be administered in a dose of 0.5 ml (25 mcg) intramuscularly one week before travel to an endemic area.The vaccine is suitable for all persons above two years of age.
b. **Oral vaccine (Ty21a oral vaccine):** Four capsules (enteric coated) should be taken orally every alternate day over one week.
   This vaccine is not suitable for children under six years of age. Booster dosage - four capsules after five years.
c. **Inactivated whole cell vaccine:** It is not recommended for use as it is not well tolerated.

Availability in India

a. Typhoral (Aventis) is available for oral use.
b. Vactyph (Zydus) is the parenteral vaccine in (0.5 ml) vial.

Precautionary Measures

Live attenuated vaccine should not be used during an attack of fever or gastrointestinal disorder nor should it be used in immune depressed states. It should be avoided if there is history of local or systemic reaction to a previous vaccination.

Drug Interaction

Oral typhoid vaccine capsules should not be taken within 24 hours of use of antibiotics and proguanil. However, there is no interaction between oral typhoid vaccine and other vaccines.

Cholera Vaccine

Cholera vaccine is useful for a short period of protection of about six months as in refugee camps. It is not recommended for travelers as it cannot prevent transmission of infection.
Two types of cholera vaccines are available:
1. *Parenteral:* Inactivated whole cell vaccine.
2. *Oral:* Live attenuated vaccine.

Schedule for Vaccination

a. Parenteral vaccine should be administered in two doses at intervals of one or two weeks. It provides protection for six months only.
b. Oral vaccine should be administered as single dose in cold or lukewarm water one hour before food or drink.

Seroconversion after oral vaccination is quick (almost 8 days) and the protective efficacy rate is 82 to 100 percent but the protection lasts for six months only.

Precautionary Measures

Vaccination should be avoided for children less than two years of age.

It should not be undertaken during an attack of fever, gastrointestinal disease and in immunocompromised individuals and pregnant women. Interval between oral typhoid vaccine (Ty21a) and oral cholera vaccine should be at least eight hours. Use of antibiotics and antimalarials should be avoided for at least seven days.

Varicella Vaccine

This vaccine is meant for adults mainly. The main beneficiaries include health care workers, immunocompromised patients and their contacts, international travelers, students and women of child bearing age.

Lyophilized vaccine containing live "oka" strain of varicella- zoster virus is available as varilix (GSK) and varipox (Zydus Biogen) in India.

Immunization schedule: The vaccine should be administered subcutaneously in two doses (0.5 ml) each at interval of eight weeks. It should be avoided in children below one year of age.

Measles-Mumps-Rubella (MMR) Vaccine

Persons born before 1957 are considered immune to measles. Those born after the above date should receive MMR vaccine. One dose of MMR provides adequate protection against mumps and rubella. It should be avoided in pregnant women and women planning to become pregnant in coming four weeks. A second dose of MMR is recommended for adults who were previously vaccinated with killed measles vaccine. Health care worker, college students and international travelers are the main beneficiaries of MMR vaccination.

Pneumococcal Vaccine

Streptococcus pneumoniae is responsible for causing pneumococcal disease particularly in elderly persons (above 65 years), very young children, and among immunocompromised individuals. Bacterial pneumonia, bacteremia and pneumonic meningitis are the conditions in which patients may become very serious. Prevention of such episodes can be achieved by vaccination at appropriate time **(Table 1.2)**.

Two types of pneumococcal vaccines are available:

1. 23- valent pneumococcal polysaccharide vaccine.
2. 7- valent pneumococcal conjugate vaccine. Both are inactivated vaccines.

Component

Polysaccharide vaccine contains purified capsular protein from 23 types of *Streptococcus pneumoniae*. However, children under two years of age show poor response to this vaccine.

The conjugate vaccine contains polysaccharide antigens from seven common types of *Streptococcus pneumoniae* conjugated to carrier protein and adsorbed into aluminium phosphate. This vaccine should not be used for children under five years of age.

Japanese Encephalitis Vaccine

Japanese encephalitis is the most common form of encephalitis in South East Asia. Almost all cases are found in children below 10 years of age. There is no specific treatment. Nearly one-third of the patients die but more than half of the survivors are left with severe debilitating neurological sequelae. Hence, prevention of the disease by use of a preventable vaccine is of utmost importance.

Currently three types of vaccines are available **(Table 1.3)**. They are:
1. Inactivated mouse brain vaccine
2. Inactivated primary hamster kidney cell vaccine
3. Live attenuated vaccine (SA-14-14-2).

Prevention Among Travelers

International travelers, students, soldiers and missionaries who have to stay for a month or longer in endemic areas particularly during transmission season should receive the protective vaccination. Even in endemic regions individuals who reside in high-risk zones like farmland, rice field, and interior areas need the vaccine. Laboratory workers working in laboratory dealing JE virus also need protection.

Table 1.2: Schedule for immunization against pneumonia-primary vaccination

Age	*Schedule*
a. 2–12 months	3 doses of conjugate vaccine 0.5 ml I.M at intervals of one month (not to be injected in buttock)
b. 12 months to 5 years	Two doses of conjugate vaccine 0.5 ml I.M at interval of at least 2 months
c. 5 years and above	Single dose of polysaccharide vaccine 0.5 ml. Adults mostly develop good antibody response by 3rd week after a single dose of vaccine. Booster doses are not routinely recommended but may be administered every 5 years for immunosuppressed individuals

Table 1.3: Dosage schedule for immunization for Japanese encephalitis

a. Inactivated mouse brain derived vaccine (Biker JE vaccine)	3 doses of 1 ml each on 0, 7 and 30 days (seroconversion nearly 100%)
b. Inactivated primary hamster kidney (PHK) cell derived vaccine note- (PHK cell linesare not approved by WHO)	1 ml subcutaneously
c. Live attenuated vaccine	Extensively used in China only

Besides above noted vaccines, some new vaccines are under development. They are verocell derived inactivated vaccine, genetically engineered vaccine and DNA vaccine.

Tomorrow's Vaccines (Vaccines Under Development)

Malaria Vaccine

Since the malaria parasite has several stages in life cycle like liver stage, blood stage (asexual stage), sporozoite and gametocytes, a vaccine needs to be fully effective against these stages. Several candidate vaccines are now under study for prevention of malaria.

The most important advance in development of malaria vaccine was made when in 1984 a vaccine was produced out of irradiated sporozoites. The genes coding for the circumsporozoite protein of plasmodium falciparum, the major surface antigen of the sporozoites were cloned and sequenced. The vaccine was tried for protection of humans but success was limited.

Liver Stage Antigen

A number of liver stage antigens (LSA) apart from CSP has been developed as vaccine candidate (LSA1, LSA3). The liver stage of the parasite is the only stage where it inhibits cell expressing HLA (human leukocyte antigen) and can therefore come under direct T-cell-mediated attack.

Some work has also been done on the development of a blood-stage vaccine. Mostly the work has been concentrated on Merozoite Surface Antigens (MSP1 and MSP2) and ring- infected erythrocyte surface antigen (RESA). A vaccine developed in Columbia (SPF 66) has been tried extensively but found to be ineffective after trial in South America, Tanzania, Gambia and Thailand.

More than 30 different antigens from different stages of life cycle of the parasite are now proposed as vaccine candidates. Transmission blocking vaccines against the gametocytes are also under development. Plasmodium vivax sporozoite vaccine is also a candidate. The vehicle for vaccine also plays an important role in immunogenicity. Antibody response is augmented if the vaccine is presented in alum or liposome. Future malaria vaccines may be multicomponent and multistage vaccines. In fact the major benefit of the vaccine may be to attenuate infection and prevent death from malaria rather than elimination of the disease.

HIV Vaccine

Investigators are working to develop a protective vaccine. However, some are busy to explore a candidate vaccine as therapeutic agent. The best vaccine should be one which can induce antibodies that can neutralize most of HIV-1 subtypes and induce T-cells to inhibit viral replication.

Some candidate envelope vaccine constructs are undergoing trial in Thailand and the result is eagerly awaited. Several phase one and two trials are under way in different regions. It may be long time before phase three trials are completed.

Japanese Encephalitis Vaccine Under Development

The following vaccines are under development for prevention of Japanese encephalitis.

a. ***Vero cell derived inactivated vaccine:*** This vaccine is under development and study in Japan, South Korea, Taiwan and China.
b. ***Genetically Engineered Vaccine (Chimeri Vax):*** It is a new live attenuated vaccine. It uses a reliable flavivirus- yellow fever 17-D as a live vector for the envelope genes of the S-14 -14 -2 virus. The early clinical trials show a promising future. The available results indicate that a single dose will provide life-long immunity against JE.
c. ***DNA Vaccine:*** It is designed to immunize against multiple flavivirus. The efficacy and immunogenicity are still to be fully determined.

Besides the vaccines discussed above, few other vaccines are also under study. They include rotavirus vaccine, cytomegalovirus vaccine, gonococcal vaccine, leprosy vaccine and toxoplasma vaccine.

Combination Vaccines

These vaccines contain antigens of multiple strains of some infectious agents causing the same disease. These vaccines can reduce the number of pricks, number of visits and decrease the cost of vaccination. Currently following combinations are available:

Hepatitis A + hepatitis B DPT + Hib

DPT+ Hepatitis B DPT + Killed polio

DPT+ Killed polio + Haemophilus influenza B (Pentavirus)

Efforts are in progress to combine as many more vaccines as possible.

BIBLIOGRAPHY

1. Anders RF, Saul A. Malaria vaccines. Parasitol today 2000;16:444-7.
2. Challenges. Adolesc Med 2000;11:211-24.
3. Clyde DF, MC Carthy VC, Miller RM. Hornick RB Specificity of protection of man immunized against sporozoite-induced malaria. Am J Med Sci 1973;266:398-401.
4. Medicine update: Assoc. Physician. India. Ed BK Sahay 2006 Vol 16.
5. Shetty NP, Shetty PS. Epidemiology of disease in tropics In: Cook GC, Zumla A (Eds). Manson's Tropical Diseases. 22nd edn. Saunders Elsevier London 2009.pp.19-34.
6. Shlim D, Solomon T. Japanese encephalitis: Vaccines for travelers: exploring the limits of risks. Clin Infect Dis 2002;35:183-8.
7. Smith D, Inskip-Paulk E. Adolescent Infectious Disease.
8. WHO position paper. Typhoid Vaccines: weekly epidemiological record 2000;75:257-64.

2

Chapter

Disaster-related Communicable Diseases: Management and Prevention

JK Dutta

Natural disasters affect some part of the globe or other almost every year. This is a major cause of concern for health services in affected regions. Outbreak of communicable diseases in particular demands emergency measures. Preparedness is the key component in disaster management.

Definition

Disaster is defined as a serious disruption of the functioning of a society causing widespread human, material or environmental losses including loss of life. This disruption is on a scale sufficient to warrant an extraordinary response from outside the affected community or area (WHO, 1995).

Types of Disasters (Table 2.1)

Disasters may be natural like cyclone, hurricane, typhoon, tornadoes, flood, drought, etc. Topographical disasters include earthquake, landslide, avalanches and tsunami. Sometimes men are responsible for disasters like nuclear or biological and chemical warfare as well as terrorism by extremists. Nearly 60% of major epidemics occur in Asia Pacific region. Out of 430 disasters recorded in 1980 to 1989, 172 disasters were recorded in India.

Table 2.1: Types of disasters

Natural	*Manmade*
A. Meteorological Hurricanes,tornadoes, typhoon, flood, drought, famine, heat and cold wave	1. Nuclear, biological, chemical warfare 2. Terrorism
B. Topographical Earthquake, landslides, avalanches, tsunami	3. Road, rail or aviation accidents 4. Fire 5. Civil strife or conflict
C. Environment	

Communicable Disease Outbreak in Disaster Setting

Following major natural disasters were recorded in India in recent years. In 2004, there was tsunami which affected Andhra Pradesh, Tamil Nadu, Kerala, Pudicherry, Andaman and Nicobar Islands, following which there was focal outbreak of measles in coastal Tamil Nadu. In the same year, flood affected Assam, Bihar and Gujarat where sporadic cases of diarrhea were recorded. Following the earthquake that occurred in Bhuj, Gujarat in 2001, sporadic cases of waterborne diseases were recorded. Soon after the super cyclone in Orissa in 1999, outbreak of leptospirosis was recorded there.

Post-Disaster Communicable Diseases (Table 2.2)

Water-borne and food-borne disease outbreaks occur usually in weeks following the disaster. However, vector-borne disease outbreaks are recorded later after four weeks or more.

In post-disaster setting water-borne diseases include cholera, viral hepatitis, typhoid and dysentery. Malaria, dengue, acute encephalitis is the common vector-borne diseases which break out after the disaster. Other diseases like measles, meningitis and leptospirosis may be recorded in some areas. Loss of human life is very high due to earthquake, landslides and epidemics. According to United Nations, at least 25000 deaths were caused in the world due to disasters in 2001 alone.

Control of Communicable Diseases in Disaster Setting (Table 2.3)

Control rooms must be set-up at state and district level. Efforts should be made to identify the source of water contamination which should be rectified. Chlorination of water should be encouraged (chlorine tablets may be used). Patients suffering from any communicable disease should be adequately treated in a well equipped center. Oral rehydration should be vigorously encouraged in areas where there is an outbreak of cholera or other water-borne diseases. Mosquito breeding sites must be treated with insecticides. Bed net and mosquito repellants may be used for personal protection. Measles vaccine should be used if there is outbreak. All fever cases should receive initial treatment for malaria. Mosquito breeding can be prevented by not accumulating empty tyres, tubes, empty coconut-shells in and around house.

Table 2.2: Post-disaster communicable diseases and their mode of spread

Diseases	*Mode of spread*
A. Acute gastrointestinal diseases–cholera, enteric fever, viral hepatitis	Water-borne
B. Malaria, dengue, acute viral encephalitis	Vector-borne
C. Others–measles, meningitis, leptospirosis	Person to person contact with infected body secretions or fomites

Table 2.3: Control of post-disaster communicable diseases

Do's	*Donot's*
1. Drink safe water (boiled or chlorinated)	1. Do not drink unsafe water
2. Keep food items covered when hot	2. Do not eat cut fruits
3. Wash hands properly before and after eating	3. Do not defecate indiscriminately
4. Use mosquito bed nets or mosquito repellants	4. Do not allow water to accumulate
5. Arrange adequate treatment for all fever and diarrhea cases	5. Do not store old tyres, tubes in which water may accumulate
6. Vaccinate and revaccinate as required against preventable communicable diseases	
7. Report outbreak of communicable diseases to health authorities for appropriate action	

Public health officials have a vital role in effective control of epidemics who should exercise adequate surveillance.

Laboratory Support

Adequate laboratory support is essential to identify the nature of microbial agents responsible for an epidemic following a disaster. Proper procedure should be adopted for collection and transport of samples to the laboratory. Tests which give quick result should be encouraged. Investigation kits should be made available for use of rapid response teams (RRT). Sophisticated investigations may be carried out in reference laboratories if essentially required.

In post-disaster setting several public health measures should receive top priority. It is important to maintain data on mortality and morbidity pattern of preventable communicable diseases. Safe water supply, proper sanitation, vitamin A supplement to young children, isolation and adequate treatment of sick persons are essential. Coordination between concerned sectors like state and district administration, municipal health administration, public health engineering department and agriculture sector is considered essential for this purpose failing which there may be undesired deterioration in essential services.

BIBLIOGRAPHY

1. CD Alert. Laboratory support in disaster situation 2003;9:1-8.
2. Control of communicable diseases manual. American Public Health Association. 17th edn. 2000.
3. Manual of laboratory techniques for district public health laboratories, NICD, Delhi 2004.
4. World Health Organization. Guidelines for assessing disaster preparedness in health sector. WHO/PAHO, Washington 1995.

3 Chapter Terrorism and Bioterrorism

JK Dutta

WHAT IS TERRORISM?

It has been defined as the unlawful use of force against persons or property to intimidate or coerce a government, the civilian population or any segment thereof in the furtherance of political or social objectives.

Bioterrorism

Some authorities suggest that terrorism by use of harmful chemicals, pathogenic microbes or plant or microbial toxins as weapons of terrorism should be known as bioterrorism. In the fall of 2001 United States experienced first multistate bioterrorism event with the delivery of anthrax spores in powder form through the mail.

Historical Background

In 1346 to 1347, the Mongols reportedly catapulted corpses of plague victims over the walls into Kaffa (now in Ukraine), forcing the Genoans to flee. In June 1763, during French and Indian wars, blankets and handkerchiefs from smallpox hospitals were distributed to Indians as gifts as a result of which epidemic of smallpox followed. In 1932, the Imperial Japanese Army began systematic development and testing of biological agents in Manchuria. During the years that followed-up to the end of 2nd World War, highly toxic agents like *Y. pestis, B. anthracis, Vibrio cholerae and N. meningitides* were used as weapons of bioterrorism. Nearly 3000 prisoners mostly children died during the program.

In 1984, more than 750 persons became ill with salmonellosis after eating from salad bars in some restaurants in Dallas, Oregon, USA. In March 1995, release of the organophosphate nerve agent 'Sarin' in Tokyo subway system is a clear instance of use of chemical or biological weapon against civilian population. Terrorist groups are classified as foreign, domestic or religious. Foreign terrorist groups may be state supported or independent.

Requirements of a Suitable Biological Weapon

- The pathogen should be readily available or easy to produce in large quantities.
- Should have highly lethal effect on humans.
- Appropriate aerosol size should be available.
- Should be stable in adverse environmental conditions.
- Should affect only the target population.
- Neither innocent human population nor the terrorists should be affected.
- Dissemination should be easy.

Potential Biological Agents

Three categories of agents have been identified as potential biological agents:

1. Agents that pose great threat in term of morbidity and mortality and need increased surveillance and stockpile of antidotes (antibiotic and vaccine).
2. Agents that can cause illness but require little public health preparation.
3. Agents as possible public health threats.

Category A Agents

Variola virus, *B. anthracis, Y. pestis, Cl. botulinum toxin,* F. tularensis, ebola virus and other arena viruses.

Category B Agents

Coxiella burnetti, Brucella species, vibrio cholerae, E. coli 0157: H7 *Shigella, salmonella* and others.

Category C Agents

Nipah virus, hantavirus, yellow fever, multi-drug resistant tuberculosis, yellow fever and tick-borne encephalitis virus.

Preparedness

Attack by bioterrorists is usually a local phenomenon and not a state wide event. Hence for adequate and timely response all local hospitals, clinics and health care delivery systems must have prompt preparedness to face an event. There may be sudden influx of a large number of ill patients and worried persons who should be provided adequate treatment, care and advice. Decontaminating process and infection control measures must be readily available. Timely detection and report of the first signal of an unusual outbreak is crucial. Nursing services, epidemiologist and public health administrators have a vital role to play. However, most health care facilities are poorly prepared to mount an effective response. Bioterrorism readiness plan template for health care facilities has been developed by some organizations. Bioterrorism is indeed a public health threat.

BIBLIOGRAPHY

1. Association for professionals in infection control and epidemiology. Bioterrorism readiness plan: A template for health care facilities 2000. http:/ www.apic.org/html/educ/readinow.html.
2. Center for Disease Control and Prevention. Biological and chemical terrorism: strategic plan for preparedness and response. Recommendations of the CDC strategic planning work group. MMWR 2000;40 (RR-4):5-6.
3. Henderson DA. Bioterrorism as a public health threat. Emerg Infect Dis 1998; 4:488.
4. Institute of Medicine. Chemical and biological terrorism. Research and development to improve civilian medical response. Washington DC. National Academy Press. 2000.pp.65-77.
5. Macintyre AG, Christopher GW, Eitzen E, et al. Weapons of mass destruction events with contaminated casualties: Effective planning for health care facilities. J Am Med Assoc 2000;283:242-9.
6. O' Neill JP. Terrorism briefing, In: Proceedings of the seminar on responding to the consequences of chemical and biological terrorism (No.1996-416-003.pp.120-123), Washington DC, US Government printing office.
7. Perrotta DM, Rawlings J, Eckman M. The specter of chemical and biological terrorism. Dis Prev News 1998;58(8):1-6.

Chapter 4 Travel and Recreation-related Infectious Diseases

JK Dutta

Travel is a necessity for many persons. Tourists often travel to specific destinations for religious or missionary activity, on government services (armed forces) or for business purpose. Due to increased travel facility, virtually any destination can be reached now in 36 hours of travel and many in less time. Increasingly, travel is now between developed and developing countries and vice versa. Travel may be for short period or may be long-term as for migrants and immigrants.

Travel and recreational activities are often closely inter-linked. Many people travel for the specific purpose of recreation whereas for others recreation is a part of the travel. Travel between tropical and temperate countries is also on the increase. It is estimated that nearly 30 to 75% of travelers to tropical and subtropical countries report some health problem.

TRAVEL

Several factors are responsible for acquiring infection during or at the end of travel. Unusual and adventurous activities like cave exploration, contact with animals, and eating unusual local foods may provide opportunities to acquire different types of infections. Walking on the road barefooted, sleeping without mosquito net and in an environment which allows exposure to rats often provide opportunities for different infections to occur.

In Asian countries places of pilgrimage and religious gathering often provide ample opportunities to acquire emerging as well as re-emerging infections. In 1987 religious pilgrims to Mecca became infected with epidemic strain of group A *Neisseria meningitides* from whom the disease spread to sub-Saharan Africa where it caused epidemics.

Migrants or immigrants may travel to safer places at the time of turmoil or disaster and bring with them infectious diseases which are endemic in their native countries. Migrants and immigrants as well as inmates of refugee camps are at special risk because they are malnourished, stressed and exposed to insanitary environment. In 1994 there was an outbreak of cholera in Zaire in refugee camps following the movement of Rwandan refugees to Zaire.

RUNWAY MALARIA

Malaria may be acquired during brief stops at airport in endemic malaria areas or due to bite by infected mosquitoes that had been imported to non-endemic country by air. Cargo handlers and customs officers of the aircraft are at special risk. In one study live mosquitoes were detected in 12 out of 67 aeroplanes that arrived at Gatwick airport in London. In 1986 mosquitoes numbering 150 were detected in 27 airplanes that arrived at Nairobi airport. The mosquitoes are carried in passenger or cargo hold as well as in wheel bays.

In cruise ships also, sometimes diseases due to different pathogens are observed due to consumption of contaminated food and water purchased locally. Gastroenteritis is the predominant illness in these patients.

Legionnaire's disease caused by *Legionella pneumophila* has been reported to be associated with travel. Recent reports have described such outbreak among cruise ship passengers who used a whirlpool spa. In 1994 there was an outbreak of *Legionella* disease in USA among 50 passengers who used the same cruise ship.

Travel-related anthrax was reported by a peculiar mode of infection. Once a traveler from USA brought home a camel hair saddle to Pakistan and gave it to a 12-year-old girl. Later she developed a large carbuncle due to cutaneous anthrax. During travel some persons may purchase food from street vendors and may suffer from diarrhea due to cholera or other infectious pathogens. Gnathostomosis caused by a nematode was acquired in Acapulco, Mexico after eating poorly cooked or raw fish particularly as "coviche". Leptospirosis was acquired by traveler to Borneo in 2000 due to contamination of open sores and leech bites. Coccidioidomycosis was acquired by some persons from USA in Mexico presumably due to dust exposure.

RECREATION

Different types of recreations may expose persons to animals, pets during hunting and camping. Some cases of *E. coli* 0157:H7 infection has been reported in Pennsylvania and Washington among visitors petting zoo and farm animals. Lyme disease may spread due to exposure to vectors of the disease during walking in forest areas. Tourists who walk barefooted or lie in bare body on sand may sometimes develop cutaneous larva migrans due to hookworm. Many people keep some exotic reptile as pets like turtle, snakes and lizards. Over 90% of reptiles carry *Salmonella enterica* which may cause gastroenteritis or meningitis in children. Home gardening may sometime be hazardous. *Legionella longbeachae* associated pneumonia has been reported due to contaminated potting soil.

BIBLIOGRAPHY

1. Center for Disease Control and Prevention. Exposure of passengers and flight crew to *Mycobacterium tuberculosis* on commercial aircraft 1992-1995, MMWR 1995;44:137-40.
2. Moore PS, Reeves MW, Schwartz B, Gellin BC, Broome CV. Intercontinental spread of an epidemic group A *Neisseria meningitides* strain. Lancet 1989;2: 260-3.
3. Rojas - Molina N, Pedraza - Sanchez S, Torres - Bibian B, et al. Gnathostomosis: An emerging food borne zoonotic disease in Acapulco, Mexico, Emerg Inf Dis 1999;5:264-6.
4. Smith L. The case of the camel hair carbuncle: Patient Care 1995;29:138-9.
5. Tremblay A, Mclean JD, Gyorkos T, et al. Outbreak of cutaneous larva migrans in a group of travelers. Trop Med Int Hlth 2000;5:330-4.
6. Ward L. *Salmonella* perils of pet reptiles. Commun Dis Publ Hlth 2000;3:2-3.

5 Chapter Transfusion and Transplantation Transmitted Infectious Diseases

JK Dutta

The ability to transmit infectious diseases by transfusion of blood and blood products depends on a variety of factors which include the pathogenesis of the infecting organism, its prevalence in blood donor population, ability to persist in a host, as well as the status of recipient's immunity. HIV is a potent example of transfusion transmitted infection. Besides several other viruses, recently concern has been expressed about potentiality of tick-borne infections like *Borrelia burgdorferi* (Lyme disease), *Ehrlichia chaffeensis, Babesia microti,* etc. Various parasitic agents like *Plasmodium vivax, P. falciparum, Trypanosoma cruzi* can also be transmitted by blood transfusion.

In current years transplantation of solid organs and vascular tissues is an important mode of therapy in some cases of end organ failures. In Germany three out of six persons who received transplants of solid organs from an infected donor developed rabies.

Transfusion-related Emerging Diseases

After blood transfusion, some infections which can develop are variant Creutzfeldt - Jakob disease (vCJD), Bovine spongiform encephalopathy (BSE) and CJD are currently noteworthy emerging diseases. Because of widespread prevalence of vCJD in Britain and Western Europe stringent restrictions on blood donation have been enforced in USA. In the last few years a number of viral agents have been identified as potential for emerging diseases transmitted via blood transfusion. These include HIV, Human-T lymphotropic-virus (HTLV-1), HTLV-11, hepatitis C, human herpesvirus 8, hepatitis G or GB virus, herpes virus 6, and putative hepatitis-linked T T Virus. The risk of transmission has been estimated as follows: HTLV-11: 1 in 6, 77,000 blood units transfused, HTLV-1: 1 in 6, 41,000, HCV: 1 in 1, 03,000 and HBV: 1 in 63,000.

Transplantation Transmitted Emerging Diseases

Xenotransplantation poses a potential risk of transmission of zoonotic diseases from animal to man. The porcine endogenous retroviruses are particularly worrisome. Particular concern is about the viruses that can cross species barriers. Pigs are now considered to be a major source of organs and tissues for transplantation in children.

Though strictly speaking rabies being a century old disease is not an emerging disease but some recent modes of spread are indeed unique. The disease is now transmitted from man to man via organ transplantation. In 2004, four patients developed rabies in USA following transplantation of organs like liver, kidney and vascular tissues. In Germany, three persons who received transplants of lung, kidney, kidney/pancreas from a common donor died of rabies.

In late December 2004, a woman died of undiagnosed rabies in Germany. Six persons received organs after her death for transplantation. Out of them three persons who had received lung, kidney, kidney/pancreas transplants developed rabies. Diagnosis of rabies was confirmed in the donor and some of the recipients by laboratory investigations carried out in the Bernhard Nocht-Institute for Tropical Medicine in Hamburg and the Konsiliarlabor for Rabies, University Clinic in Essens Institute of virology.

There is also a solitary report of transmission of West Nile virus through solid organ transplantation. These reports underscore the potential for transmission of infectious diseases in organ transplant recipients. Hence, it is essential that very scrupulous care is taken for recruitment of infection-free donors. All recruiting agencies and organizations should exercise maximum care in this respect. All appropriate investigations should be carried out to exclude the possibility of existence of any infection which may endanger the recipient's life after transplantation.

BIBLIOGRAPHY

1. Allain JP. Emerging viruses in blood transfusion. Vox. Sanguinis 2000;78(suppl 2): 243-8.
2. Breitschwerdt EB, Kordick DL. Bartonella infection in animals: carriership, reservoir potential, pathogenicity, and zoonotic potential for human infection. Clin Microbiol Rev 2000;13:428-38.
3. Center for Disease control and prevention. Update: Clostridium novyi and unexplained illness among infecting-drug users. Scotland, Ireland, and England. April-June 2003 MMWR 2000;49:543-5.
4. Chamberland ME, Alter HJ, Bruch MP, Nemo G, Ricketts M. Emerging infectious disease issues in blood safety. Emerg Inf Dis 2001;7(3 suppl):552-3.
5. Dumber JS, HOM. Risk factors and approaches to infections in transplant recipients. In: GL Mandell, JE Burnett, RE Dollin (Eds). Mandell, Dougles and Bennett's principles and practice of infections diseases. Philadelphia, Churchill Livingstone 2000;3126-36.
6. Dutta JK. Organ Transplant Related Rabies. In: Human Rabies. 1st edn. 2005. pp.37-40. Sradha publication. Balasore.
7. Gunzburg WH, Salmons B. Xenotransplantation. Is the risk of viral infections as great as we thought? Mol Med Today 2001;6:199-208.

8. Kahan BD, Clark JH. Transplantation of solid organs. In: MM Frank, FK Austen, HN Claman, ER Unanue (Eds). Samter's immunologic disease. Boston, Little Brown 1995;11:1495-509.
9. Mabey DCW. Chlamydial infections. In GT Strickland (Ed). Hunter's Tropical Medicine and Emerging infectious diseases. 8th edn. 2000.pp.349-51. Philadelphia, WB Saunders.
10. Maguina C, Gotuzzo E. Bartonellosis: New and old Inf Dis Cl N. America 2000;14:1-22.
11. Stoler MH, Bonfiglio TA, Steigbigel RT, Pereira M. An atypical subcutaneous infection associated with acquired immune deficiency syndrome. Am J Cl Pathol 1983;80:714-8.

6 Chapter
Hospital Infection: Prevention and Control

JK Dutta, Madhumala Giri

Infection is an established cause of human death. Though death is inevitable, the cause of death varies. Hospital infections cannot be totally eliminated but can be controlled. Man has learnt from experience - which forms the basis of modern day hospital infection control programs.

The administrative authorities in hospitals should establish high standard for control of infection and to prevent new infection. Following are few frightening lines quoted from the book, "Secret agents: The menace of emerging infections" authored by Madeline Drexler.

"Infection is an inescapable part of life. All creatures feast upon other creatures and in time are feasted upon in a kind of eschernesque food chain. When humans are the meal, we call it infectious disease".

Statistics in USA indicate that compared to previous decade, morbidity and admission rates due to infections has increased by 58% and mortality by 22% in this decade (excluding HIV/AIDS).

Infectious microorganisms love two things (a) overcrowding (b) poor sanitation. We should know how to live in symbiosis with microorganisms without producing morbidity. Research should be directed towards reducing premature death from any infection.

In earlier years Louis Pasteur established the "germ theory" of disease and Lister proved the benefits of disinfectants and aseptic surgical technique. Nightingale, Semmelweis, Holmes and others established the principle of hygiene.

Infection Control Program in USA

In 1970's the Center for Disease Control and Prevention in USA began the nation wide project: Study of the efficacy of nosocomial infection control (SENIC). After a decade the study showed that in approximately 33%, reduction was achieved in urinary tract infection, surgical wound infection, pneumonia and bacteremia in hospitals where the control program was active.

Problems and Control of Hospital Infections in India

In India the hospitals are overcrowded. Due to shortage of beds patients are compelled to sleep on the floor. In most places the environment is unhygienic. The ward boys, ward *ayas* and other servants barely understand the basic principles of hygiene.

Management of hospital waste is a major problem in India. Incineration is not permitted in many parts of the country due to production of toxic chemicals such as dioxin. Laundry can be an easy source for transfer of infection.

The health care workers have great role and responsibility to achieve success in hospital infection control program. Infection control committees should be set up in each hospital consisting of a physician, surgeon, a senior nurse and a microbiologist. Data collection, surveillance and enforcing good infection control practices are the important functions of the committee. "Infection prevention week" should be held at least once in a year by the committees when the whole staff engaged in the program may be galvanized.

It is equally important that the health care workers employed in health institutions must be free from any communicable disease. Similarly, person-to-person transmission of infection must be prevented by isolation and "barrier nursing" of persons suffering from potentially transmissible diseases.

Luckily the incidence of hospital infection is on an average 5 to 10% with 1% mortality. However, it must be emphasized that nosocomial infection is a serious problem which must be fought tactfully.

BIBLIOGRAPHY

1. Bennett JV, Brachman PS. Hospital Infections. 4th edn. Philadelphia. Lippincoot-Raven 1998.
2. Burke JP. Infection Control - A problem for patient safety. N Engl J Med 2003; 348:651-5.
3. Egglmann P, Pitter D. Infection Control in ICU. Chest 2001;120:2059-93.
4. Secret Agents. The menace of emerging infections. Madeline Drexler. Joseph Henry Press.
5. VIcent JL. Infection in adult intensive care unit. Lancet 2003;361:2068-76.

Section B

Infectious Diseases

7 Chapter

Ehrlichiosis

JK Dutta

Since mid 1970s more than 20 new tick-borne infectious diseases have been identified in man. Ehrlichiosis came to attention in 1987. Ehrlichiosis is named after Paul-Ehrlich, the former German Physician who was born in 1854 in Upper Silesia in Eastern Germany. At Breslau University he described the mast cell by a new staining technique. In recognition of his work on "immunity" he was awarded Nobel Prize at the age of 54 which he shared with Metechnikoff of the Pasteur Institute of Paris. He died in August 1915 in Frankfurt.

Ehrlichia are gram-negative bacteria in the family Rickettsiaceae. The species which infect man are *E. chaffensis, E. senretsu, E. canis, E. phagocytophila* and *Eequi* (HGE agent), and *E. ewingii.*

In man ehrlichiosis is manifested in two clinical forms, Human monocytic Ehrlichiosis and Human Granulocytic Ehrlichiosis. Co-infection with Lyme disease or Babesiosis has been observed in some patients **(Fig. 7.1)**.

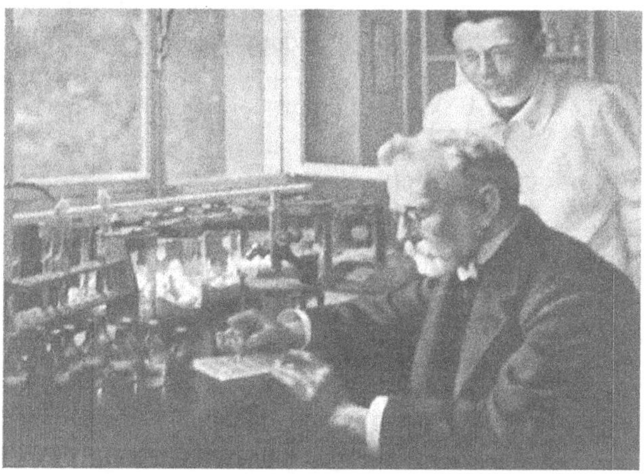

Fig. 7.1: Ehrlich: Chemotherapy is launched

Human Monocytic Ehrlichiosis (HME)

Clinical Features

It is caused by *E. chaffeensis.* The transmission to man occurs through a Lone store tick, *Amblyomma americanum.* Monocytes are the main target cells.

Incubation period is about eight days. The disease has a severe course in children in whom death may occur. Fever is the most frequent complaint which is observed in nearly 97% patients. Headache, myalgia, nausea, vomiting and unexplained cough may be the other manifestations.

Complications

Complications may be severe. Septic shock like syndrome, adult respiratory distress syndrome, meningoencephalopathy and hemorrhage may develop as complications. Severe form of opportunistic infection may be evident in some cases. In nearly 62% cases the disease has a severe course.

Diagnosis

Leucopenia is frequently observed. Initially there may be lymphopenia followed by neutropenia. In nearly 70% patients, thrombocytopenia is evident. However, morulae are rarely seen in peripheral blood.

Bone-marrow examination reveals hypercellularity with noncaseating granuloma. Hepatic aminotransferase level is usually elevated. PCR is also a helpful method for diagnosis which shows amplification of *E. chaffeensis* nucleic acid. Serological diagnosis indicates previous infection if there is four fold rise in antibody level in paired sera.

Treatment

Doxycycline 100 mg orally or intravenously twice daily is highly effective. Alternatively tetracycline 250 to 500 mg orally every six hours may be used. Most patients are cured after a short course of antibiotic therapy for 3 to 5 days. Tick bite should be avoided by proper clothing for prevention.

Human Granulocytic Ehrlichiosis (HGE)

It is caused by *E. phagocytophila* which is transmitted by lxodes scapularis and also by lxodes pacificus ticks.

Clinical Manifestation

Incubation period is 4 to 8 days. The peak incidence occurs in May-July. Fever, myalgia, nausea, vomiting and unexplained cough are the usual symptoms. There is an influenza-like illness with case fatality less than 1%.

Complications

Toxic shock syndrome, adult respiratory distress syndrome, and opportunistic infections are the notable complications. In elderly persons and children the complications are usually more severe.

Diagnosis

In peripheral blood there is leucopenia and thrombocytopenia. On examination of bone marrow, morulae may be detected which will indicate a positive parasitic diagnosis. PCR on EDTA - anticoagulated blood collected before start of antibiotic therapy is a highly sensitive method of diagnosis. Positive serology indicates past infection.

Treatment

Doxycycline 100 mg twice daily orally is very effective for treatment. Rifampicin can be effectively used for pregnant women. Levofloxacin and ciprofloxacin are the other alternative drugs which have been found suitable. No vaccine is available for prevention.

BIBLIOGRAPHY

1. Buller RS. *Ehrlichiae ewingii*, a newly recognized agent for human ehrlichiosis. N Engl J Med 1999;341:148-50.
2. Dumler JS, Bakken JS. Human ehrlichiosis: Newly recognized infection transmitted by tick. Annu Rev Med 1998;49:201-3.
3. Dutta JK. Ehrlichiosis. Indian Drug Review 2005.pp.50-1.
4. John Talbot. Biographical history of Medicine. Grunet Stratton. London 1970.
5. Mc Quiston JH, Paddock CD, Holman RC, Childs JE. The human ehrlichiosis in the United States. Emerg Infect Dis 1999;5:635-42.
6. Rikisha Y. The tribe *Ehrlichiae* and ehrlichial disease. Microbiol Rev 1991;4: 288-9.
7. Taylor JP, Betz TG, Fishbein DB, et al. Serological evidence of possible human infection with *Ehrlichiae* in Texas. J Inf Dis 1998;158:217-20.

8

Chapter

Bartonella Infections

JK Dutta

Bartonella was first recognized by Barton in 1908. It was formerly called "*Rochalimaea*". *Bartonella* genus has increased rapidly. Now the genus includes 16 species. At least five species are known to cause disease in man. They are *B. bacilliformis, B. henselae, B. quintana, B. elizabethae* and *B. claridgeae.* Bartonella are aerobic, fastidious, gram-negative bacteria.

As yet the term bartonellosis (Carrion's disease) is applied to infections caused by *B. bacilliformis, B. henselae* and *B. quintana* are transmitted by cat scratch and body louse (responsible for trench fever) respectively. In AIDS patients they cause biliary angiomatosis, peliosis hepatitis and systemic infections.

BARTENELLOSIS (CARRION'S DISEASE)

The disease has two distinct phases:

1. Acute febrile hematinic phase (Oroya fever)
2. Eruptive phase with cutaneous lesions (verruga peruana)

Carrion a medical student infected himself with tissues from verruga peruana in 1885. He died after developing Oroya fever. It was thus proved two disorders are linked.

Clinical Features

Oroya Fever

The classical features of Oroya fever caused by the infection are insidious onset of fever with malaise, pain in lower joints and macrocytic anemia with reticulocytosis. Superinfection with *Salmonella typhimurium* may prove fatal. In some patients, after 3 to 4 months of fever the disease progresses to verruga peruana stage (localized bartonellosis).

Verruga Peruana

It is the localized manifestation of bartonellosis which develops after a long time following Oroya fever. It is usually a sequel of Oroya fever but may arise spontaneously in some patients.

The miliary eruptions are most marked on face and extensor surfaces of extremities. A pink macule which first appears becomes nodular. The nodules may develop on mucous membrane of mouth, oesophagus, stomach, intestine, bladder, uterus and vagina. So there may be episodes of bleeding from above sites. Frequently Oroya fever and verruga stages co-exist.

Management

The treatment of choice for Oroya fever is chloramphenicol + ß-lactam agent or ciprofloxacin. Verruga peruana is treated with rifampicin or streptomycin.

Cat-scratch Disease

Cat-scratch disease is caused by *Bartonella henselae*. The definitive host is cat or rarely the dog. The infection is transmitted to man mostly by bite of domestic cat and less commonly from dogs.

Clinically there is enlargement of lymph nodes draining the sites of bite or scratch. A small papule develops followed by enlargement of lymph nodes draining the area which may resolve spontaneously over several months. Usually no treatment is required.

In bacillary angiomatosis (BA) there is a vascular, nodular or papular growth. Lesions may also develop in gastrointestinal tract, larynx and bones. In bacillary peliosis (BP) cystic blood-filled spaces develop in liver, spleen, sometimes in lymph nodes. The victims are almost always patients with AIDS. Bacillary angiomatosis (BA) and bacillary peliosis (BP) are both caused by *B. quintana* and *B. henselae*, both BP and BA can be effectively treated with erythromycin or doxycycline.

Trench Fever

The disease was described in the First World War. The term "trench fever" was coined by Hunt and Rankin who described 30 cases. His and Werner described the disease in 1916 in German troops in the Eastern Front. McNee et al. wrote a detailed description from the Western Front.

Etiology

The etiological agent is *Bartonella quintana*. The infection is transmitted by body louse. Rubbing louse feces into scarified skin is the most common mode of transmission to man. Bite by louse is a very uncommon mode of spread.

Clinical Features

The incubation period is 7 to 98 days. In experimental trench fever, classically the patient develops a sudden attack of influenza-like illness. There is high fever with retro-orbital headache and pain in limbs. Severe persistent anterior tibial pain is the classical but unexplained feature. Probably the pain is neurological in nature. There is an erythematous rash which is transient. After 2 to 8 days the fever subsides but relapses again. Some patients have a prolonged episode of relapsing and remitting fever. Splenomegaly is not unusual. *B. quintana* may cause retinal artery occlusion and peripapillary angiomata with severe loss of vision. *B. quintana* is now recognized as an important cause of endocarditis.

Diagnosis

In blood culture, growth is slow. However, diagnosis can be made by culture, by serological study and histologically with specific PCR on infected tissue like heart valve. The organism can be seen by acridine organ staining of cultured blood and the DNA can be amplified for a positive culture.

Management

The organism is sensitive to many antibiotics *in vitro*. Mild cases can be treated with doxycycline. Patients with bacteremia should be treated with doxycycline and gentamicin. Replacement of heart valve may be required in some cases of endocarditis.

BIBLIOGRAPHY

1. Adal KA, Cockerell CJ, Petri WA Jr. Cat scratch disease, bacillary angiomatosis and other infections due to Rochalimaea. N Eng J Med 1994;330:1509-15.
2. Breitschwerdt EB, Kordick DL. Rochalimaea infection in animals: carriership, reservoir potential, pathogenicity, and zoonotic potential for human infection. Clin Microb Rev 2000;13:428-38.
3. Conrad DA. Treatment of cat-scratch disease. Curr Opin Ped 2001;13:56-9.
4. English CK, Wear DJ, Margileth AM, Lissner CR, Walsh GP. Cat scratch disease: isolation and culture of the bacterial agent. JAMA 1988;259:1347-52.
5. Kerkhoff FT, Bergmans AMC, Van der zee, Roghova A. Demonstration of *Bartonella* grahami DNA in ocular fluids of a patient with neuroretinitis. J Clin Microbiol 1999;37:4038.
6. Kerkhoff FT, Ossewarde JM, de Loos WS, Rothova A. Presumed ocular bartonellosis. Br J Ophthalmol 1999;83:270-5.
7. Koehler JE. *Bartonella*: A morning human pathogen. In: WM Scheld. Anmstrong J and JM Hughes (Eds): Emerging infect, 1998 (147-163). Washington DC. ASM press.
8. Liang Z, Raoult D. Species specific monoclonal antibodies for rapid identification of *Bartonella quintana*. Clin Diagn Lab Immunol 2000;7:21-4.
9. Maguina, Gotuzzo E. Bartonellosis New and old. In Dis Clin N Am 2000;14: 1-22.
10. Mehanna D, Peck N, Arnot R, Solano T, Sheldton D. Cat scratch disease presenting as splenic abscess. Aust NZ J Surg 2000;70:622-4.
11. Peters D, Wigand R. Bartonellaceae-Bact. Rev 1955;19:150-9.
12. Ricketts WE. Clinical manifestations of Carrion's disease. Arch Intern Med 1949;84:751-81.

13. Salgado CD, Weisse ME. Transverse myelitis associated with probable cat-scratch disease in a previously healthy pediatric patient. Clin Infect Dis 2000;31:609-11.
14. Schultz MG. Daniel Carrion's experiment. N Engl J M 1968;278:1323-6.
15. Thompson PK, Vaphiades MS, Saccente M. Cat-scratch disease presenting as neuroretinitis and peripheral facial palsy. J Neuro-ophthalmol 1999;19:240-1.

9 Chapter

Escherichia Coli 0157: H7

JK Dutta

In September 1999, ten children developed bloody diarrhea and were hospitalized in Albany, New York. They had attended the Washington County fair that was held in the last week of August. By the middle of September, 921 persons were ill due to diarrhea. They all had attended the fair. Stool cultures from 116 persons yielded *E. coli* 0157:H7. Two persons died which included a 3-year-old girl and a 79-year-old man. The patients developed diarrhea due to infection from an unchlorinated well water.

Characteristics of the Organism

Escherichia coli is a gram-negative, nonspore forming, rod-shaped bacteria of the family Enterobacteriaceae. The pathogenic strains that can cause illness are categorized as enterohemorrhagic, enteroaggregative, enterotoxigenic, enteroinvasive, enteropathogenic and diffuse-adherent based on virulence mechanisms. *E.coli* 0157:H7 was first described as a human pathogen in 1982 by Center for Disease Control and Prevention during two outbreaks of hemorrhagic colitis.

Clinical Features

The incubation period is 1 to 14 days from the day of exposure. Most patients develop diarrhea with or without blood, severe abdominal pain, and vomiting. Hemolytic uremic syndrome (HUS) and thrombotic thrombocytopenic purpura may develop as complication which is followed by death. HUS is the most significant clinical complication which may be observed in 60 to 70% patients. In 1992, there was a large outbreak of *E. coli* 0157:H7 infection in Washington, Idaho, California and Nevada in USA due to undercooked hamburgers served in a restaurant. Overall this infection is estimated to infect about 21,000 persons in USA annually.

Prevention

Safe water supply and high standard of personal hygiene are important as preventive measures. Food-handlers should follow strict hygienic measures and they should have proper awareness about the mode of spread of the infection and the dreadful consequences.

BIBLIOGRAPHY

1. Center for disease control. Isolation of *E-coli* 0157:H7 from sporadic cases of hemorrhagic colitis-United States. MMWR 1982;34:581-5.
2. Center for Disease control and prevention. Outbreak of *Escherichia coli* 0157:H7 infections among children associated with farm visits-Pennsylvania and Washington 200. MMWR 2001;50:293-7.
3. Mead PS-Griff in PM *Escherichia Coli* 0157:H7 Lancet 1998;352:1207-12.
4. Weightman NC, Kirby PJG. Nosocomial *Escherichia coli* 0157 infection. J Hosp inf 2000;44:107-11.

10 Chapter

Antibiotic Resistant Enterococci and Drug Resistant *Streptococcus Pneumoniae*

JK Dutta

ENTEROCOCCI

Enterococci are categorized as "emerging infections" because they have developed resistance to ampicillin and vancomycin. Organisms in the genus *Enterococcus* are facultatively anaerobic, gram-positive cocci. Enterococci are normal inhabitants of the intestinal tract of man and animals. There are at least 17 species in the genus which include *Enterococcus faecalis* and *E. faecium*. They are prevalent in many areas in the world. Contaminated food products and colonized animals act as reservoir of infection. Enterococci which are resistant to vancomycin include *E. faecalis*, *E. faecium*, *E. gallinarum* and *E. durans*.

Clinical Illness

Urinary tract infection is the most common clinical illness. Bacteremia, endocarditis, pelvic infection, neonatal sepsis, meningitis may also develop. Respiratory infection is very uncommon.

Treatment

Serious infection caused by enterococci requires combination therapy with penicillin and an aminoglycoside (gentamicin, streptomycin). Recently quinupristin-dalfopristin (a streptogramin combination) and linezolid have been recommended for treatment of vancomycin-resistant *Enterococcus faecium*.

DRUG RESISTANT *STREPTOCOCCUS PNEUMONIAE*

Streptococcus pneumoniae (*pneumococcus*) is the most frequent cause of pneumonia, meningitis, otitis media, sinusitis, arthritis, peritonitis, endocarditis and septicemia in different parts of the world.

Clinical Illness

The organism was named as *Pneumococcus* in 1886, *Diplococcus pneumoniae* in 1920 and finally as *Streptococcus pneumoniae* in 1974. It is a gram-positive, catalase negative lancet shaped bacteria which replicates in pairs or chains and is usually encapsulated. It is a facultative anaerobe. There are 90 different serotypes. The highest risk of infection is noticed among immunosuppressed persons (congenital agammaglobulinemia), lymphoma, aplastic anemia, infants and malnourished children. Death usually occurs in elderly, immunocompromised and asplenic patients who may develop meningitis and bacteremia due to infection before death.

Drug Resistance

The first case of antibiotic resistant *S. pneumoniae* was reported in 1964. By now more than 20 strains showing penicillin resistance have been identified. On world wide consideration the drug resistance rate is about 40 to 70%. In fact resistance has been recorded to all antibiotics except vancomyin. However, reports of resistance to vancomycin do exist. Elderly persons above 65 years of age, children under two years and HIV infected persons are at high-risk of infection. Use of inappropriate antibiotic dosage is a contributing factor for development of drug resistance. A newer oral drug telithromycin has been found to be as effective as vancomycin.

BIBLIOGRAPHY

1. Center for Disease Control and Prevention. Diagnosis and management of food-borne illness. A primer for physicians. MMWR. 2001;50 (RR - 02):1-69.
2. Cetinkaya Y, Falk P, Mayhall CG. Vancomycin-resistant enterococci. Clin Microbiol Rev 2000;13:686-707.
3. D'Agata EMC, Green WK, Schulman G, et al. Vancomycin resistant enterococci among chronic haemodialysis patients: A prospective study of acquisition. Clin Infect Dis 2001;32:23-9.
4. Musher *D. Streptococcus pneumoniae*. In Mandell G, Bennett J, Dolin R (Eds) Princ Pract Infect Dis 5th edn. 2000.pp.2128-47. Philadelphia: Churchill Livingstone.
5. Whitney CG, Farley MM, Halder J, et al. Increasing prevalence of multidrug resistant *Streptococcus pneumoniae* in the United States. New Engl J Med 2000;343:1917-24.

Chapter 11 Salmonellosis

TK Dutta, V Mukta

INTRODUCTION

Salmonellosis is a major cause of bacterial enteric illness in both humans and animals. Specific Salmonella serotypes cause a spectrum of illnesses which can be broadly divided into typhoidal and nontyphoidal Salmonella infections.

History

Salmonella is named after the pathologist Salmon who first isolated *Salmonella choleraesuis* from porcine intestine. Typhoid fever was so named because its symptoms and signs resembled typhus. William Jenner distinguished typhoid in 1850 by the presence of the pathological evidence of enlargement of Peyer's patches and mesenteric lymph nodes. Wilson proposed the term enteric fever in 1869, as it is an intestinal infection. In 1880 Eberth described bacillus typhous in the histological sections of mesenteric lymph nodes and spleen of persons dying of typhoid fever in 1880. Gaffky first cultured *Salmonella typhi* in 1884. In 1896 Widal described the Widal reaction and Wright and Pfeifer introduced the vaccination against typhoid.

Epidemiology and Public Health

Salmonellosis is a global problem, but now patients with typhoid and paratyphoid fever are mainly found in the developing nations where the sanitary conditions are poor. World wide, 16 million cases of typhoid fever are estimated to occur annually with six lakh deaths. Typhoid and paratyphoid fevers are endemic in the Indian subcontinent, South east and Far East Asia, the Middle East, Africa, Central and South America. While the incidence of typhoid fever has decreased, the incidence of nontyphoidal Salmonellosis has increased in the developed countries. Nontyphoidal *Salmonella* infections are the most common cause of food-borne disease outbreaks in developed countries. The proportion of typhoid to paratyphoid fevers is about 10:1. Paratyphoid B and C are rare. Enteric fever is most common in the 5 to 20 years age group. Typhoid fever occurs in two epidemiological types. First is the endemic or residual typhoid fever that occurs throughout the year, though seasonal variations may be apparent. The second is the epidemic typhoid which is usually water or foodborne. Food handlers or cooks who become carriers are important cause of infection. Mary Mallon (Typhoid Mary) was one such cook, who over a period of seven years caused at least seven outbreaks affecting over 200 people.

The Pathogen

Salmonella is a genus of the family Enterobacteriaceae. Based on a high degree of DNA similarity, all *Salmonella* isolates are included in a single species, *S. choleraesuis*. This species further has seven subspecies based on DNA similarity and host range. Subspecies 1 has most of the serotypes typed into one of more than 2300 serovars according to somatic O, surface Vi and flagellar H antigens. For simplicity, most *Salmonella* serotypes are named for the city in which they were defined and the serotype is often used as the species designation. Strictly *Salmonella typhi* should be written as *Salmonella* subspecies *choleraesuis serovar typhi.*

Salmonella are facultative anaerobic gram-negative rods, 2 to 3 by 0.4 to 0.6 µm in size, motile by peritrichous flagella. They produce acid on glucose fermentation, reduce nitrates and do not produce cytochrome oxidase. *Salmonella typhi* does not produce gas on sugar fermentation.

Salmonella can be isolated in the microbiology laboratory using a number of low-selective media (MacConkey agar, deoxycholate agar), intermediate-selective media (*Salmonella-Shigella* [SS] agar, Hektoen [HE] agar), and highly selective media (selenite agar with brilliant green). Individual isolates can then be distinguished by serotyping bacteriophage typing, and genotyping.

S. typhi, S. paratyphi A, and S. schottmuelleri produce enteric fever, *S. Choleraesuis* produces septicemia or focal infections. *S. typhimurium* and *S. enteritidis* produce gastroenteritis.

Antigenic Analysis

Salmonella are classified on the basis of two surface antigens, somatic O antigen and flagellar H antigen **(Table 11.1).** According to Kauffman-White classification system, nine serogroups (A through I) are defined by O antigens. All members of a serogroup carry the different minor O antigens. Serotypes within serogroups are differed by the H antigens. An individual serotype may carry one or more types of H antigens, referred to as phase 1 or phase 2. A third type of antigen, the virulence or Vi antigen is present on *S. typhi* and occasionally on *S. paratyphi C.*

Table 11.1: Antigenic analysis by the kauffman-white scheme of the organisms causing typhoid and paratyphoid fever

	O antigen Group	*O antigen*	*H antigen Phase 1*	*H antigen Phase 2*	*K antigen*
S. paratyphi A	A	1,2,12	a		-
S. schottmuelleri	B	1,4,5,12	b	1,2	-
S. hirschfeldii	C	6,7	c	1,2	Vi
S. typhi	D	9,12	d		Vi

Flow chart 11.1: Pathogenesis of *Salmonella* infection

Ingestion of contaminated food or water

↓

Salmonella cross the acid barrier in the stomach

↓

Traverse through the M cells in the Peyer's patches of small intestine

↓

Salmonella are phagocytosed by macrophages and multiply within them

↓

Salmonella spread to reticuloendothelial tissues via lymphatics

↓

Salmonella drain from thoracic duct into the blood stream

↓

Bacteremia

Pathogenesis and Pathology

All salmonella infections begin with ingestion of organisms in contaminated food or water **(Flow chart 11.1)**. The infectious dose varies from 103 to 106 colony forming units.

Immunology: Typhoid fever induces both humoral and cellular immune responses. It has been proposed that immunization with the oral typhoid vaccine (Ty 21a) may be mediated by antibody dependent cellular cytotoxicity involving IgA antibodies against *S. typhi* and CK4 + T-cells.

Infections in man: Clinical manifestations in man can be described as follows **(Table 11.2)**:

Table 11.2: Clinical diseases caused by *salmonella*

Disease	*Enteritis (S. typhimurium and enteritidis)*	*Septicemia (S. choleraesuis)*	*Enteric fever (S. typhi)*
Onset	Abrupt	Abrupt	Insidious
Incubation period	<48 hours	Variable	10–20 days
Fever	Low	Rapidly rising	Gradually rising
Duration of disease	<5 days	Variable	Few weeks
Early constipation	–	–	+
Diarrhea	+	–	Occurs late
Blood cuture	–	+	+ve in early stage
Stool culture	+	+/–	+ve in late stage

Typhoidal Salmonellosis

Enteric fever- Typhoid fever, paratyphoid fever
Chronic carrier state

Nontyphoidal Salmonellosis

Gastroenteritis
Bacteremia and vascular infection
Localized infection

Enteric Fever

Causative organism- *Salmonella typhi* causes typhoid fever, *Salmonella paratyphi A, Salmonella paratyphi B (S. schottmuelleri)* causes paratyphoid fever.

Typhoid Fever

Incubation period: 10 to 20 days (range 3–56 days), depending on the number of organisms ingested and immune status of the host.

During first week of illness flu-like prodromal illness, headache, anorexia, cough, myalgia, diarrhea and abdominal pain occur. There occurs fever (101.8 degrees F–104.9 degrees F), which increases daily in a stepwise fashion but may be remittent or sustained. Patient is toxic, apathetic and may be delirious. Less than 25% cases have relative bradycardia. Rose spots, which are blanching, faint salmon colored maculopapular rash, 2 to 4 mm in size may be seen on the abdomen and chest. Patient has coated tongue, tender abdomen and moderate hepatosplenomegaly. Rhonchi, crackles may be heard over the lung bases.

Typhoid state: Patient develops neuropsychiatric manifestation like muttering delirium, picking at clothes, muscle twitching, psychosis and confusion in the third week of illness. This is called as typhoid state. It is seen in 10% of the patients. Patient may also develop stiff neck, stupor and focal neurologic deficit.

Fever remains in the second week, and then comes down by spontaneous lysis. Temperature returns to normal by the end of the fourth week.

Complications: Intestinal perforation and hemorrhage are late complications which occur in the third or fourth week of illness. Rare complications of typhoid fever are pancreatitis, hepatic and splenic abscesses, endocarditis, pericarditis, nephritis, pneumonia, parotitis, arthritis, osteomyelitis, cerebellar ataxia and schizophrenia. 10 to 20% relapses after initial recovery and antibiotic treatment.

Carrier State

- Those patients who shed *Salmonella* in feces for three weeks to three months after clinical cure are called convalescent carriers.
- Those who shed the bacilli for more than three months but less than one year are called temporary carriers.
- 1.5% becomes chronic carriers, who shed the bacteria in the stool or urine for more than one year.
- Incidence of chronic carriage is higher in women, persons with hepatic infection with *Opisthorchis sinensis*, gallstones and gastrointestinal malignancies.

Paratyphoid fever: The illness is milder, of shorter duration and the complications are infrequent.

Nontyphoidal Salmonellosis

The causative organisms are *S.typhimurium* and *S.enteritidis*. They are usually acquired from multiple animal reservoirs. There is marked seasonal variation in its occurrence. It peaks in summer in temperate countries and in rainy season in tropical countries due to increased incidence of food poisonings.

The source of infection is eggs, poultry, undercooked meat, unpasteurized dairy products and contact with infected exotic pets like lizards, snakes.

Clinical Syndromes

Gastroenteritis

Clinical Features

- Incubation period: 6 to 48 hours after consumption of contaminated food/water.
- Fever (100.5 to 102.2 degrees F), resolves within 72 hours.

- Moderate volume, non-bloody, secretory diarrhea occurs which resolves within 3 to 7days.
- Chronic carrier state is rare (<1%).
- Severe illness occurs in the neonates, elderly and the immunosuppressed.
- Rarely mimics appendicitis or inflammatory bowel disease.

Bacteremia

- Protracted hectic fever with chills, anorexia, weight loss .
- Gastrointestinal symptoms, rose spots, leucopenia are absent.
- *S. choleraesuis, S. paratyphi, S. dublin, S. typhi* are four serotypes commonly associated within USA.
- Bacteremia follows enterocolitis in 1 to 4% of adults.

Endovascular Infection

- 5 to 10% of bacteremic persons develop localized infection.
- *Salmonella* have propensity for infecting vascular sites. If >50% of three or more blood cultures are positive, an endovascular infection should be suspected.
- *Salmonella* endocarditis (incidence 0.2–0.4%) produces rapid and extensive valvular destruction and perforation. Risk factor—pre-existing valvular heart disease. Mortality is ~ 70%.
- Myocardial abscess, purulent pericarditis, mural and major embolism are common complications of *Salmonella* endocarditis.
- Arteritis should be suspected in elderly with back pain/ abdominal pain, preceded by diarrhea.
- Arteritis can be associated with mycotic aneurysms, ruptured aneurysms, vertebral osteomyelitis. *S. choleraesuis* is the most common isolate.

Pulmonary Infection

- Predisposing factors—pre-existing lung or pleural abnormality, elderly, immunocompromised states, cardiac disease.
- Pneumonia, lung abscess, pleural effusion, bronchopleural fistula.
- Mortality ~ 25 to 60%

Central Nervous System Infection

- Meningitis and its sequelae in neonates (<4 months old) - ventriculitis, obstructive hydrocephalus, brain abscess. (incidence- 0.1–0.9%). Mortality ~ 40 to 60%

Osteomyelitis

- Predisposing factors—sickle cell anemia, hemoglobinopathies, diabetes, systemic lupus erythematosus, corticosteroid therapy, pre-existing fractures.

- Bones affected—femur, tibia, humerus, lumbar vertebrae, spine, costo-sternal junctions.
- Incidence <1%

Arthritis

- Pyogenic arthritis complicates 0.2 to 0.3% of hospitalized Salmonellosis cases.
- More often in infants, those with prosthetic joint implants.
- Joints involved—knee, hip, shoulder, sacroiliac joints.
- Hematogenous spread is cause.
- Reactive arthritis (Reiter's syndrome) can follow Salmonella gastroenteritis, more often those with HLA-B27 antigen.

Genitourinary Tract Infection

a. Predisposing factors—urolithiasis, structural abnormality, malignancy, immunosuppresion.
b. Cystitis, pyelonephritis.
c. Testicular/ovarian abscess, epididymitis/salpingitis.
d. Incidence 0.6%

Intra-abdominal Infections

- Predisposing factors- anatomical abnormalities of hepatobiliary systems, gallstones, malignancy, sickle cell disease.
- Hepatic, splenic abscess
- Cholecystitis
- Mortality ~ 10%

Enteric Fever Diagnosis

Investigations

For isolation of the causative agent, blood, urine, stool, bone marrow, gastric or intestinal secretions, rose spots, mononuclear cell platelet fraction can be used. A positive culture for *S. typhi, S. paratyphi* is obtained in more than 90% of the cases if blood, bone marrow and intestinal secretions all are performed. The sensitivity of blood culture alone is only 50 to 70%, probably because of the small quantities of *S. typhi* (i.e. <15 organisms/ml) that are typically present in the blood of patients of typhoid fever. The sensitivity of bone marrow culture is 90% and unlike blood culture is not reduced by up to 5 days of prior antimicrobial therapy. Stool cultures are more often positive in children (60%). *Salmonella* can be isolated from stool and urine of chronic carriers for periods longer than 1 year.

- *Blood culture:* Since the onset of febrile phase is associated with bacteremia, blood culture is often positive in the first week of illness. By third week, it is found in 50% of patients. Blood clot cultures yield a higher rate of isolation as the bactericidal action of the serum is obviated.

- *Stool culture:* Typhoid bacilli are most easily isolated from the feces between the third and the fifth week of illness.
- *Urine culture:* may be positive after the second week of illness.

Widal test is a serological test to detect antibody against *S. typhi*. In this test the patient's serum is tested by tube agglutination for its titers of antibodies against H, O and Vi antigens of *S. typhi* and *S. paratyphi*. It is diagnostic, if a four-fold or more rise in the antibody titer can be demonstrated in two samples collected at a gap of 10 to 14 days. Serologic tests for Vi antigen are useful to detect long-term carriers as they have high antibody titer to this antigen.

Serotype is identified by the slide agglutination test. Coagglutination method has been tried to detect the *Salmonella* antigen in the blood. ELISA has been attempted for detecting Vi antigen in the urine. However the diagnostic value of these tests is yet to be established.

DNA probes for *S. typhi* have been developed but are not commercially available.

Bacteriophage typing, Biotyping, Plasmid typing are used to establish the epidemiology of the disease.

Diagnosis of Nontyphoidal Salmonellosis

Enterocolitis: The diagnosis of *S. enterocolitis* requires isolation from stool. Polymorphonuclear leukocytes are present in stool.

Bacteremia: Blood cultures. Once bacteremia is documented, it is important to determine if it is high grade (>50% of three of more of blood cultures positive); if so, endovascular infection is possible and further evaluation is needed.

Blood leukocyte counts are reduced in enteric fever, remain normal in enterocolitis and are elevated in localized suppuration.

Treatment

Enteric Fever

Chloramphenicol was introduced in 1948, given in the dose of 500 milligrams four times a day, it produced defervescence and relief of symptoms in 3 to 4 days, reduced the case fatality from 10 to 15% in the preantibiotic era to 1 to 4%. Its major disadvantages are:

- It does not reduce the relapse rate.
- It does not cure the convalescent excretor or the chronic carrier.
- It causes aplastic anemia in 1 in every 10,000 to 50,000 patients.
- It is not useful to treat R-Plasmid-mediated, chloramphenicol resistant strains of *Salmonella typhi*.

After 1970, ampicillin (1 gram orally every 6 hourly) and trimethoprim-sulfamethoxazole (TMP-SMX; one double strength tablet twice daily), became the mainstay of treatment, Because of the recent emergence of multidrug resistant strains of *S. typhi*, including plasmid mediated resistance to ampicillin and trimethoprim, the efficacy of these drugs has also diminished. Epidemiologically *Salmonella typhi* strain resistant to any two known antibiotics usually effective against (typhoid fever) is called as multidrug resistant strain. Thus either quinolones or third generation cephalosporins are currently recommended for empirical antibiotic treatment **(Table 11.3)**. Ciprofloxacin, though safe, may rarely cause pancytopenia and bone marrow depression. First and second generation cephalosporins and aminoglycosides are ineffective for treating Salmonellosis. Short course therapy with ofloxacin (10–15mg/kg divided twice daily for 2–3 days) appears to be simple, safe and effective treatment of uncomplicated multidrug resistant typhoid fever, when strain is susceptible to Nalidixic acid. Quinolones are contraindicated in children and pregnant women as it caused cartilage damage in animal studies. In 1993, Nalidixic acid resistant strains (NARSTs) were isolated, which had mutations involving DNA gyrase. Thus, when NARST strain is suspected, a higher dose of ciprofloxacin or longer duration of ofloxacin is recommended.

In cases with severe typhoid fever (i.e. with associated delirium, obtundation, stupor, coma, shock) and with a positive culture for *S. typhi* or *S. paratyphi*, dexamethasone treatment should be considered. A single dose of 3 mg/kg followed by eight doses of 1 mg/kg given every 6 hours has been tried with good results.

Chronic Carriers

Treatment with oral amoxicillin TMP- SMX, ciprofloxacin, norfloxacin for six weeks is effective in eradicating chronic carriage in 80% cases.

Table 11.3: Antibiotic therapy for typhoid fever

Antibiotic	*Dosage*
First Line	
Ciprofloxacin	500 mg PO bd for 7–10 days
Ofloxacin	10–15 mg/kg in 2 divided doses for 3 days
Ceftriaxone	1–2 gm IV/IM daily for 7–10 days
Cefixime	200–400 mg as single or in 2 divided doses for 10–14 days
Furazolidone	7.5 mg/kg PO qid for 2 weeks
Alternative (NARST)*	
Azithromycin	1 gm PO daily for 5 days
Ciprofloxacin	10 mg/kg PO bd for 10days (750 mg bd in adults)
Ofloxacin	10–15 mg/kg in 2 divided doses for 7–10 days.

*Nalidixic acid resistant *S. typhi*

- Without cholelithiasis—oral ampicillin or amoxicillin-100mg/kg/ day + probenicid 30 mg/kg/day, or trimethoprim sulfamethoxazole two tablets twice daily for three months.
- With cholelilithiasis—surgery + antimicrobials as above.
- With schistosomiasis—treat schistosomiasis first.

Vaccines

Three vaccines are currently available:

1. "Heat killed, phenol extracted whole cell vaccine.
   Administration-two 0.5 ml subcutaneous injections >4 weeks apart; booster every three years."
   Adverse reactions—fever, malaise, pain or swelling at the injection site.
2. Ty 21q, an attenuated *S. typhi* vaccine (four oral doses). Minimal age for vaccination is six years. Efficacy-29 to 96% for two years or longer.
3. Vicps-purified Vi polysaccharide from the bacterial capsule (one parenteral dose). Minimum age for vaccination is two years, Efficacy-65 to 75% for 17 months or longer. Administration-one 0.5 ml intramuscular dose, booster every two years. Adverse reaction—fever, headache, erythema or induration at the injection site.
4. Vi-rePA-Vi Polysaccharide bound to a nontoxic recombinant protein (two parenteral doses). Minimum age for vaccination six months.

Currently Ty 21a or ViCPS are being used for vaccination of travelers to endemic countries.

Nontyphoidal Salmonellosis

Rehydration with fluid and electrolyte replacement for *nontyphoidal salmonella gastroenteritis* is recommended. Antibiotics are generally not recommended except in the following situations:

- Neonates up to three months of age
- Persons older than 50 years
- Transplant recipients
- HIV patients, prosthetic joints
- Underlying sickle cell disease.

For the above patients, 24 to 48 hours of oral or intravenous antibiotics are recommended. For the immunocompromised, longer duration of therapy, 7 to 14 days may be needed.

Focal Infections or Life-Threatening Bacteremia

Empirical therapy with a third generation cephalosporin or quinolone is recommended.

- Low grade bacteremia—7 to 14 days of antibiotics
- AIDS patients with *Salmonella* bacteremia—1 to 2 weeks of antibiotics followed by 4 weeks of oral quinolones

- Relapse case—long-term suppressive therapy with quinolone or TMP-SMX
- Endovascular infection-intravenous betalactam antibiotics
- Infective endocarditis—early surgery, six weeks of third generation cephalosporin.
- Arteritis—early surgical bypass, six weeks of third generation cephalosporin.
- Chronic osteomyelitis, abscesses, urinary and biliary tract abnormality-surgical intervention.

BIBLIOGRAPHY

1. Ananthanarayan. Paniker-Enterobacteriacae III: *Salmonella*. In Paniker CKJ (Ed). Ananthanarayan and Paniker's Textbook of Microbiology. 7th edn. Orient Longman. Hyderabad 2005.pp.290-304.
2. Bhatia R, Icchpujani RL. *Salmonella*. In: Promila (Ed). Essentials of Medical Microbiology. 3rd edn. Jaypee brothers. New Delhi 2004.pp.245-53.
3. Dutta TK, Badhe BA. Ciprofloxacin induced bone marrow depression. Postgraduate Medical Journal 1999;75:571-3.
4. Dutta TK, Beeresha, Ghotekar LH. Atypical manifestations of typhoid fever. Journal of Postgraduate Medicine 2001; 47:248-51.
5. Dutta TK, James J, Jayanthi S. Correlation of clinical and hematological profiles with bone marrow response in typhoid fever. American Journal of Tropical Medicine and Hygiene 1997;57:313-6.
6. Dutta TK, Shanmuganathan C, Kanungo R, Ghotekar LH. Management of typhoid fever-An update. In API Medicine update. Editor and publisher Gupta SB, Mumbai 2002;123:1120-4.
7. Gianella RA. *Salmonella*. Mandell GL, Benett JE, Dolin R (Eds). Principles and practice of infectious diseases. 5th edn. Churchill Livingstone. New York 2000;1138-39,3251-2.
8. Hoffman SL. Typhoid fever. In Wright SG, Monath TP, Latharn MC, Keystone JS (Eds). Strickland Hunter's Tropical Medicine. 7th edn. WB Saunders. London 1998;345-66.
9. Jenkins C, Gillespie SH. *Salmonella* infections. In: Cook G, Zumla AI. Manson's Tropical Diseases. 22nd edn. Saunders. London; 2009.pp.931-42.
10. Miller SL, Pegues DA. *Salmonella* species including *Salmonella typhi*. In: Mandell GL, Benett JE, Dolin R (Eds). Principles and practice of infectious disease. Fifth edn. Churchill Livingstone. New York 2000.pp.2344-56.
11. Parry CM, Tran Tinh Hien, Dougan G, Withe NJ, Farrar J. Typhoid fever. New England Journal of Medicine 2002;347:1770-81.
12. Pegues DA, Miller SI. Salmonellosis. In: Fauci AS, Braunwald E, Kasper DL, et al. (Eds). Harrison's Principles of Internal Medicine. 17th edn. McGraw Hill. New York 2008.pp.956-62.

12 Chapter

Cholera

JK Dutta

Cholera is widely prevalent in the deltas of river Ganges and Brahmaputra in India and Bangladesh. It is also widespread in many other countries in South-East Asia and Africa. A devastating outbreak of cholera occurred in 1854 in London. At that time cholera was supposed to be caused by a fog coming from the river (''miasma''). Lord John Snow, the London anesthetist tied down the handle of the water pump of the Broad Street Pump in Soho that supplied water to the area. There was sharp decline in the incidence of new cases of cholera which proved that cholera was caused by contaminated water. There have been six pandemics in the past **(Table 12.1)**.

The current seventh pandemic has involved almost the whole world, which began in 1961.

Etiology

Classically, cholera is caused by *Vibrio cholerae* which was first recognized by Robert Koch in 1883. Vibrios are coma shaped gram-negative organisms. There are two biotypes *Vibrio cholerae* classical and *Vibrio cholerae* EI Tor. The biotype EL Tor was first recognized in 1906 in Sinai and remained confined to Sulawesi, Indonesia till 1961. Each biotype has 3 serotypes-Inaba, Ogawa, Hikojima. EI Tor biotype can hemagglutinate chicken cells.

Table 12.1: First six pandemics of cholera

Pandemic	*Period*	*Regions affected*	*Regions not affected*
1st	1817–23	Indian subcontinent, South-East-Asia, Middle East, East Africa	Europe, North Africa, America
2nd	1826–1838	Indian subcontinent, South-East-Asia, Middle East Europe, North and East Africa, America	Nil
3rd	1839–1855	All regions	Nil
4th	1865–1875	All regions	Nil
5th	1881–1896	All regions	Nil
6th	1899–1923	Indian subcontinent, South-East-Asia, Middle East Europe, East Africa	North Africa, America

It gives Voges-proskauer test positive and is resistant to polymyxin B. Classical biotype of the vibrio has reverse properties in these respects. The vibrio has both flagellar and somatic antigens. The organism is subdivided into serogroups based on the somatic O antigen. There are over 200 serogroups.

Recent studies have shown that *Vibrio cholerae* (including 01 and 0139 strains) are normal inhabitants of surface water particularly brackish water. There they survive and multiply in association with zooplankton and phytoplankton quite independently of infected human beings. Cholera vibrio 01(serogroup) has 145 phage types and 0139 (serogroup) has 5 phage types. Only 01 and 0139 serogroups can cause epidemics and even pandemic. *Vibrio cholerae* that do not agglutinate with 01 or 0139 antisera are referred to as non-01 non 0139 *Vibrio cholerae*. Previously they were termed as non-cholera vibrios. In 1992 a new 01 subgroup of *V. cholerae* caused an unusual outbreak of cholera in India and Bangladesh which was designated as 0139 Bengal. A related organism vibrio parahemolyticus and some non-cholera vibrios can occasionally cause cholera-like symptoms though most infected persons remain asymptomatic. Besides *Vibrio parahaemolyticus, V. fluvialis, V. hollisae, V. minicus, V. cholerae* non-01 (non-cholera vibrios) are sometimes responsible for causing diarrheal diseases. *Vibrio cholerae* is destroyed at 55°C in 15 minutes. Probably there is some genetic predisposition in cholera. Blood group O is associated with higher infection rate than group A. The role of H2 receptor antagonist regarding predisposition is not clearly understood.

Pathophysiology

The vibrio is noninvasive but produces an enterotoxin which causes excessive loss of fluid and electrolytes. The vibrios multiply within the lumen of the small intestine and do not invade the mucosa nor enter the portal circulation. Adherence of the vibrio to mucosa of small intestine is due to outer membrane protein and flagellar adhesion. Cholera toxin comprises of subunits-B (binding) and A (active). The binding subunit binds to a specific monosialosyl ganglioside, GM on epithelial cells of small intestine. A subunit is then able to migrate through the epithelial cell membrane. Because of ADP ribosyl transferase activity it causes transfer of ADP ribose from NAD to a GTP binding protein which regulates adenylate cyclase activity. As a result there is increase in cyclic AMP activity which inhibits sodium chloride absorption and stimulates chloride excretion. So there is excessive loss of water, sodium chloride, potassium and bicarbonates. Histological and electron microscopic appearances of small intestinal mucosa are normal.

Antibodies to enterotoxin and to O antigen are produced following the infection. Protective immunity is dependent on the immune response within the gut where both locally produced IgA and serum-derived IgG and IgM may be present. Antitoxin antibodies are produced to both A and B subunits of enterotoxin. Vibriocidal antibodies within the gut are serotype specific.

Epidemiology

The disease is closely associated with unsafe water supply to communities. Man is the only known reservoir of infection. The disease mainly spreads through contaminated food or water. In developed countries under-cooked seafood is the usual vehicle for transmission. Fecal contamination with excreta of patients suffering from the disease or those in convalescent stage is the principal mode of transmission. Overcrowding in places of pilgrimage during fairs and religious festivals used to be the usual places of outbreak in the past.

Currently biotype EI Tor is the predominant biotype in large areas in India. For EI Tor cholera the case to carrier ratio ranges from 30:1 to 50:1 whereas for classical biotype the ratio is 5:1. EI Tor biotype can survive long in the environment. Since the original outbreak in Sulawesi in Indonesia, this biotype spread in 1968 to Indian subcontinent. By 1996 it had almost completely replaced the classical biotype in India. In the Infectious Diseases Hospital in Delhi in 1974 through 1976, EI Tor biotype was isolated on culture from all the 175 cases included in the study. In another study among tribal population of Orissa conducted in 2002 to 2003, *Vibrio cholerae* 01, Ogawa was isolated in 2.5% of rectal specimens only. Only in Bangladesh the classical biotype is still persisting. In endemic regions, children in 2 to 4 years age group are the common victims. The disease has seasonal relationship also. In Bangladesh, most outbreaks are noted after monsoon. Outbreaks often follow cyclones and floods. Nosocomial infection has also been reported. In an outbreak in October 1992 in Madras, a new serotype 0139 was recognized. By December 1992, the outbreak caused by this serotype was identified in Bangladesh mostly among adults. Subsequently this serotype was isolated in outbreaks of cholera in Thailand.

Clinical Features

Incubation period is short which varies from few hours to 5 days. In patients infected with EI Tor biotype, the picture is of mild diarrhea. Many of them remain asymptomatic unlike classical cholera. In classical cholera caused by biotype 01, there is sudden onset with passage of 'rice-water' like stool. As much as 30 liters or more fluid may be passed in untreated patients in 24 hours which contain large number of vibrios. Vomiting often follows. Intense thirst, muscle cramp, hoarseness of voice develops due to dehydration. Hypomagnesimea is a known feature in patients of EI Tor cholera.

If rehydration is delayed, the patient may die of acute circulatory failure. Mortality rate depends on the promptness of rehydration. Quicker the rehydration, earlier is the relief. In 'cholera sicca' there is little diarrhea or vomiting but collapse and death follow rapidly. Some persons continue to excrete the vibrios for few weeks as 'carriers' even after clinical cure.

Complications

Acute renal failure is the most common complication in untreated patients or those who receive treatment late. Hypoglycemia may develop particularly in children. Electrolyte loss leads to hyponatremia and hypokalemia. Paralytic ileus and cardiac arrhythmia may develop due to hypokalemia. Confusion, convulsion, and coma may precede death.

Diagnosis

Laboratory diagnosis is essential when sporadic cases occur or during an extensive outbreak. Dark-field microscopy of rectal specimen will show the characteristic 'darting' movement of the vibrios. Addition of diluted 01 antisera to the slide will stop the movement if the organism is *Vibrio cholerae* 01 serotype. Culture of the specimen in thiosulphate citrate bile salt sucrose (TCBS) agar will confirm the diagnosis. Serotyping and biotyping may be carried out in reference laboratories. Sensitivity to antibiotics must be carried out for help of the clinicians. Molecular methods like PCR and DNA probes will help to distinguish different strains.

There are certain differences in properties of classical and EI Tor biotype of *Vibrio cholerae* 01 which are tabulated below **(Table 12.2)**.

MANAGEMENT

Oral rehydration is the most appropriate treatment in majority of cholera cases with mild to moderate rehydration. Glucose used in the oral solution enhances the active up-take of sodium and water. Glucose and glycine-stimulated membrane transport takes place normally in cholera as enterocyte sodium-glucose carrier system is not affected by cyclic AMP.

Oral rehydration fluid containing sodium chloride 5 gm, sodium bicarbonate 4 gm, potassium chloride 1 gm and water made up to 1 liter is widely used. A person weighing 50 kg with moderate dehydration will need 5 liters of the fluid within first four hours. It may be here worth noting the composition of cholera stool **(Table 12.3)**.

Total requirement of fluid is based on degree of dehydration which should be monitored clinically from time to time. In rural areas if glucose is not available, sucrose may be used. Sachets of prepared glucose-electrolyte solutions are available commercially. WHO recommended fluid in sachets, which are also available **(Table 12.4)**.

Home made sucrose and rice-water solution is quite effective. The constituents are readily available in almost every family in rural areas. In

Table 12.2: Differentiating properties of classical and El Tor biotypes of *Vibrio cholerae*

Property	*Classical*	*El Tor*
Chicken cell hemagglutination	Negative	Positive
Voges-Proskauer test	Negative	Positive
Polymixin B sensitivity	Sensitive	Resistant

Table 12.3: Electrolyte composition of cholera stool

	Na+(mmol/L)	*K+(mmol/L)*	*CL-(mmol/L)*	*Base(mmol/L)*
Adult	135	15	90	30
Child	100	25	50	30

Table 12.4: Composition of different rehydration solutions (oral and intravenous) (mmol/L)

Fluid	*Sodium*	*Chloride*	*Potassium*	*Bicarbonate*	*Glucose*
WHO ORS	90	80	20	30	111
Dhaka	133	98	13	48	0
Ringer's solution	130	109	4	28	0

patients with severe dehydration and shock, intravenous fluid should be promptly used. Intravenous glucose may be used for children who often develop hypoglycemia as a complication of cholera.

Oral rehydration therapy has revolutionized the management of cholera. A cholera patient might lose as much as 8 to 10 % of body fluid within 3 to 4 hours of onset and hence vigorous rehydration therapy is essential.

Initial phase: Aim is to replace water and salt already lost by oral route in moderately severe cases.

Maintenance phase: Aim is to replace ongoing losses of fluid and electrolytes.

World Health Organization (WHO) recommended that oral rehydration solution (ORS) can be used for both phases in nearly 80 to 90% cholera patients. It should contain sodium chloride 3.5 g, sodium bicarbonate 2.5 g, potassium chloride 1.5 g, glucose (anhydrous) 20 g and water to make 1 liter of solution.

Quantity: 50 to 100 ml of ORS per kg body weight within first 4 hours.

In the maintenance phase, loss of stool should be replaced by required volume of oral solution. Vomiting is no contraindication to use of oral solution. An adult weighing 60 kg with 10% loss of fluid will require 6 liters of ORS for initial rehydration.

Clinical assessment of dehydration by "Dhaka Method" is a useful procedure in clinical practice **(Table 12.5)**.

Table 12.5: Clinical assessment of dehydration

Signs	*Some dehydration*	*Severe dehydration*
General appearance	Restless, irritable	Lethargic or unconscious
Eyes	Sunken	Very sunken and dry
Tears	Absent	Absent
Mouth and tongue	Dry	Very dry
Thirst	Thirsty, drinks eagerly	Drinks slowly or not able to drink
Skin Pinch	Goes back slowly	Goes back very slowly

Some dehydration is present if the patient has sunken eyes, dry mucosa and feels thirsty (or skin turgor is reduced or patient is irritable/less active). Such a patient needs rehydration with oral rehydration salt solution (ORS) with frequent assessment.

Severe dehydration: Two or more of above signs and very sunken, dry eyes or absence of tear or very dry mouth and tongue are indicators of severe dehydration. Please note that tears are relevant signs only for infants and children. The skin pinch is a less useful sign in patients with marasmus or obesity.

If a patient is lethargic/comatose or unable to drink or has uncountable pulse/absent radial pulse, in addition to other signs of some rehydration, he should be categorized as a case of 'severe dehydration'. Such a patient will need rehydration with intravenous fluid and ORS with more frequent reassessment.

Ringer lactate solution is an appropriate fluid for intravenous use. 'Dhaka solution' is also a suitable fluid for intravenous therapy. Ringer lactate (Hartman's solution) does not contain adequate potassium. So potassium chloride (10–15 ml/L) can be added separately. Normal saline is not effective but may be used under compelling circumstances if other suitable solutions are not available. Oral solution should be administered as soon as the patient can drink.

'Cholera Cot' is a suitable device for treatment of patients in which fluid loss can be conveniently measured. The cot has a central hole through which stools are passed into a calibrated bucket. Intake/output chart should be maintained at the bedside which will be helpful to calculate the requirement of fluid.

Antimicrobial Agents

In all confirmed cases of cholera a course of antibiotic is advisable to sterilise the intestinal tract of vibrios and prevent further spread in the community. WHO recommends tetracycline or chloramphenicol 500 mg every 6 hours for 3 days; others believe that the period of therapy for three days only is not adequate. Where facilities permit, stool culture should be carried out daily until 3 consecutive cultures become negative when the patient can be discharged from the hospital. This practice was followed in the Infectious Diseases Hospital in Delhi.

Oxytetracycline 500 mg every 6 hours orally for 3 days is recommended for adults. Doxycycline in a single dose of 300 mg with food is quite effective. Erythromycin 500 mg every 6 hours for 3 days is a suitable alternative. It is the drug of choice for children who need 12.5 mg/kg every 6 hours for 3 days. Tetracycline should be avoided in pregnant women and children less than 8 years of age.

Trimethoprim-sulfamethaxazole is equally effective. Two tablet (each tablet containing trimethoprim 80 mg and sulfamethoxazole 400 mg) may be administered twice daily for three days for adults. Children will need correspondingly lower dosage.

Emerging drug resistance is an ever-present concern. For adults with cholera in areas where tetracycline resistance is prevalent, ciprofloxacin either in a single dose (30 mg/kg, not to exceed a total dose of 1 g) or in a short course (15 mg/kg bid for three days, not to exceed a total daily dose of 1 g) is a clinically effective substitute.

Antimicrobial Resistance

Antibiotic resistance by cholera vibrio was unknown before 1977. Later conjugative - plasmid- mediated multiple antibiotic resistance of *V. cholerae* 01(MARV) was recognized first in Tanzania and then in Bangladesh. In recent years, resistance to tetracycline, ampicillin, kanamycin, streptomycin, sulphonamides, trimethoprim and gentamicin have been reported in cholera endemic countries. However, in an earlier study by the author, trimethoprim-sulphamethoxazole (TMP-SMX) was found to be significantly better than tetracycline and chloramphenicol ($p<0.001$).

Resistance of 0139 strains to sulphonamide, trimethoprim, chloramphenicol and low level of streptomycin has been recorded. Fluoroquinolone-resistant strains of *V. cholerae* have been lately reported.

Preventive Measure

During the epidemic prompt treatment of patients and suitable disposal of excreta and other infected materials are the priorities. Drinking water must be boiled and cooled before use in all households. Purchase of fish and other perishable items must be stopped. All persons handling the patients and their excreta must wash hands with soap and water.

The whole-cell injectable cholera vaccine is no longer recommended because of low efficacy. New oral cholera vaccines provide substantial protection against the disease. A killed oral vaccine (Dukoral) consists of killed *V. cholerae* along with the cholera B subunit. Therefore it stimulates both antibacterial and antitoxic immunity. The other oral vaccine (Orochol) consists of an avirulent mutant of *V. cholerae*, strain CVD 103 HgR which is given as a single dose lyophilised vaccine.

BIBLIOGRAPHY

1. Alam AN, Alam NH, Ahmed J, Sack DA. Randomized double blind trial of high dose doxycycline for treating cholera in adults. BMJ 1990;300:1618-21.
2. Barua D, Paguio AS. ABO blood groups and cholera. Ann Hum Biol 1977;4: 489-92.
3. Barua D. The global epidemiology of cholera in recent years. Proc R Soc Med 1972;65:423-8.
4. Cholera working group. International centre for Diarrhoeal Diseases Research, Bangladesh. Large epidemic of cholera like disease in Bangladesh caused by *Vibrio cholerae* 0139 synonym Bengal. Lancet 1993;342:387-90.
5. Cohen MB, Giannella RA, Bean J, et al. Randomized controlled human challenge study of the safety, immunogenicity and protection efficacy of a single dose of Peru-15, a live attenuated oral cholera vaccine. Infect Immun 2002;70:1965-70.
6. Dutta JK, Santhanam S, Misra BS, Ray SN. Effect of Trimethoprim-sulphamethoxazole on vibrio clearance in cholera (EL Tor): A comparative study. Tans Roy Soc Trop Med Hyg 1978;72:40-2.
7. Dutta JK. EL Tor cholera in India. J Assoc Physicians Ind, 1993;41:315.
8. Hart CA, Shears P. Bacterial enteropathogens. In: Cook GC, Zumla A (Eds). Manson's Tropical Diseases. 22nd edn, Saunders Elsevier; 2009.pp.911-29.
9. Islam A, Bardhan PK, Islam MR, Rahman M. A randomized double blind trial of aspirin versus placebo in cholera and non-cholera diarrhoea. Trop Geogr Med 1986;38:221-5.
10. Sack DA, Sack RB, Nair GB, Siddique AK. Cholera (Seminar) Lancet 2004; 363:223-33.
11. Sack RB, Siddique AK, Longini IM Jr, et al. A 4-year-old study of the epidemiology of vibrio cholerae in four rural areas of Bangladesh. J Inf Dis 2003;187:96-101.
12. Tacker CO, Lasonsky G, Nataro JP, et al. Initial clinical studies of CVD 112 *Vibrio cholerae* 0139 live oral vaccine: a safety and efficacy against experimental challenge. J Infect Dis 1995;172:883-6.
13. Waldor MK, Keusch GT. Cholera and other vibrios In: Fauci AS, Braunwald E, Kasper DL, et al. (Eds). Harrison's Principles of Internal Medicine 17th edn. Mc Graw Hill, New York;2008.pp.968-72.
14. Waldor MK, Makalanos JJ. Emergence of a new cholera pandemic, molecular analysis of virulence determinants in *Vibrio cholerae* 0139 and development of a live vaccine prototype. J Infect Dis 1994;170:278-83.
15. World Health Organization Guidelines for cholera control. WHO/CDD/SER. 80.4 Geneva, WHO;1993.
16. World Health Organization. Potential use of oral cholera vaccine in emergency situations. Report of a WHO meeting. WHO/cds/csr/edc/99.4 Geneva, WHO; 1999.

13 Chapter
Plague: The Current Scenario

JK Dutta

There have been three well documented pandemics of plague in the world in the past, first pandemic Justinian pandemic 542-767 AD, second pandemic began in central Asia (1347), third pandemic began in China (1894). In the 14th century 'Black Death' swept across Europe killing nearly one-third of the population.

In India there were about ten million deaths by 1919. During 1960s and early 1970s there was a resurgence of the disease in Vietnam. In USA there were 27 deaths from plague during the period 1982 through 1996. All cases were confirmed there by Center for Disease Control and Prevention. Nearly 80% cases were in New Mexico, Arizona and Colorado. The disease is endemic in many countries in the globe even now. In 1992, 603 cases of plague were reported to World Health Organization.

Current Global Scenario

Plague is endemic in China, Laos, Mongolia, Myanmar and India. During 1962 to 1972, thousands of people died in Vietnam due to the disease. Sporadic cases are reported from Peru and Bolivia. An outbreak of pneumonic plague was reported from Ecuador in 1998. There are several foci of plague within the Russian Federation and Kazakhstan. Wild rodent plague is prevalent in Western half of USA. In 1990s human plague recurred in several African countries.

Scenario in India

In *'Bhagwat Purana'* there is mention about plague in India. The most devastating outbreak was recorded during the last pandemic in 1898. Natural foci of the disease exist in several states like Andhra Pradesh, Gujarat, Himachal Pradesh, Karnataka, Maharashtra and Tamil Nadu. During the period 1967 to 1993, there was no case of plague in the country. However after a lapse of about 28 years the disease re-emerged in August 1994 in Maharashtra state.

In September 1993, there was a devastating earthquake in Latur and Osmanabad districts of Maharashtra state. The inhabitants of Mamla village of Beed district and neighboring villages left their home out of panic and shifted to temporary shelters. However food grains were stored in their old habitation. Due to easy availability of food grains there was enormous growth in population of rats in the area. There was an epizootic among the rats, due to which death of rats was noticed by the villagers in August 1994. Soon after, there was an outbreak of bubonic plague in the village and adjoining areas. Some cases of pneumonic plague were also reported from Surat in Gujarat state. The disease gradually spread to Delhi, Varanasi, Madhya Pradesh, Karnataka and Uttar Pradesh where cases of pneumonic plague were reported. A total of 876 cases with 54 deaths were reported in this outbreak.

Very recently, pneumonic plague has been reported from Shimla district of Himachal Pradesh in February 2002. A person contacted infection in the forest which spread to others out of whom four died. Diagnosis was confirmed by several tests in laboratory. In some of them, fluorescent antibody test and bacteriophage lysis test for *Y. pestis* were positive. Molecular tests confirmed the presence of *Y. pestis* specific Pla and Fi genes. DNA finger print also had identity with known sequence of plague bacilli. Four more persons became ill after visit to the hospital where confirmed cases of plague were admitted. One out of them died on February 20, 2002.

Etiology

Plague is caused by *Yersinia pestis*. The organism was successfully isolated first by Alexandre Yersin in Hongkong in 1894. Since then it is known after his name. Previously it was known as *Pasteurella* pestis. It is a small, gram-negative, non-sporing and non-motile oval bacillus with rounded ends and convex sides. Because of bipolar staining it has a closed '*safety pin*' like appearance.

Epidemiology

Ground squirrels, rabbits, hares are the common natural reservoirs of infection. Sometimes old carnivores and domestic cats also transmit the disease. *Rattus rattus* and *Rattus norvegicus* are the most important reservoirs.

Rat fleas transmit the infection from plague infected rats to humans which results in an outbreak of human plague. Xenopsylla cheopis and Xenopsylla basiliensis are the important fleas responsible for transmission of plague.

Clinical Manifestations

The disease manifests in different forms namely bubonic plague, pneumonic plague, septicemic plague, cutaneous plague and meningeal plague.

Bubonic Plague

Incubation period is short, 2 to 6 days. There is sudden onset of fever, bodyache followed by tender, painful swelling of lymph nodes resulting in a bubo. Usually the bubo appears in the groin but sometimes in axilla or other areas also.

Pneumonic Plague

Fever, chest pain, cough, hemoptysis and respiratory difficulty are the main manifestations. It spreads rapidly among the contacts by droplet infection. Mortality is very high.

Septicemic Plague

There was an outbreak of septicemic plague in New Mexico during 1980 to 1984. In USA outbreak during 1970's, septicemic plague accounted for 11% of cases. The patient becomes actually ill with high fever, rigor, skin rash and prostration. Abdominal pain, nausea, vomiting are more frequent. *Y. pestis* may be detectable in peripheral blood smear. The patient develops shock and death follows soon.

Meningeal Plague

Primary meningitis due to plague is rare. Usually inadequately treated or untreated patients of bubonic plague develop meningeal manifestations. There is fever, bodyache and neck stiffness. Cerebrospinal fluid examination shows neutrophilic leukcocytosis. Mortality is higher than in uncomplicated bubonic plague.

Other Forms of Plague

Tonsillar and cutaneous forms are rare. In tonsillar plague, the tonsil becomes inflamed with cervical lymphadenopathy and parotid swelling. In cutaneous form, pustules, eschar may develop or there may be erythema gangrenosum. Some patients remain asymptomatic while organisms may be present in their throat.

Laboratory Diagnosis

In bubonic plague, fluid may be aspirated and smear may be examined after staining with Wayson, Giemsa or Gram stain for bipolar stained coccobacilli. In pneumonic and meningeal forms, throat swab, sputum or CSF may be processed in the same way. Blood and other appropriate samples should be sent to laboratory for culture to confirm the diagnosis which should be collected before start of antibiotic therapy. Serological tests are also available which are useful for diagnosis in culture-negative cases. Immunofluorescence antibody tests, enzyme immune assay and radioimmune assay may be used for diagnosis.

Differential Diagnosis

Bubonic plague with bubo in inguinal region should be differentiated from lymphadenopathy due to venereal infection like secondary syphilis, lymphogranuloma venereum and granuloma inguinale.

Toxoplasmosis, infectious mononucleosis, *Streptococcus pyogenes* or *Staphylococcus aureus* infections should be excluded if lymphadenopathy involves cervical or other lymph nodes.

Treatment

Response to antibiotic therapy is dramatic. Penicillin is not effective in this disease.

Streptomycin

It has remained the drug of choice for past several years. It should be used in dosage of 30 mg/kg per day in two divided doses intramuscularly for 10 days. Ototoxicity and renal function impairment are the main adverse reactions.

Tetracycline

It should be given in dosage of 4 to 6 gm in divided doses daily in first 48 hours. Subsequently when fever subsides, the drug should be continued in dosage of 15 mg/kg every 6 hours for 10 days. In seriously ill patients the drug may be used intravenously.

Chloramphenicol

This drug is particularly useful in patients with meningeal manifestation. After a loading dose of 25 mg/kg it should be continued as 60 mg/kg in 4 divided doses daily till the patient improves.

Cotrimoxazole

It is useful particularly for children. One teaspoonful of syrup every 12 hours may be used for children under 5 years of age.

Even a single antibiotic therapy is highly effective in treatment of plague. So there is no need for combination of drugs. Relapses are extremely rare. Failure of beta- lactam antibiotic has been reported in one study in murine *Y. pseudotuberculosis* infection.

Prophylactic Measures

Chemoprophylaxis is recommended for persons exposed to cases of plague. Tetracycline, doxycycline or trimethoprim sulfamethoxazole (TMP-SMX) may be used for this purpose. Tetracycline 1 to 2 g daily or doxycycline

100 to 200 mg daily may be used orally. TMP-SMX 1.6 g daily orally will be required for an adult. Ciprofloxacin in a dose of 500 mg twice daily has also been suggested lately. For immunoprophylaxis, a formalin killed plague vaccine may be used. For an adult, 0.5 ml is to be injected subcutaneously followed by 1 ml after 7 to 14 days. Booster doses are required every 6 months. Medical and public health workers and laboratory personnel who deal with infected material and samples should be vaccinated.

Soon after the identification of *Y. pestis* as causative organism, a crude vaccine was developed by Waldeman Haffkine in Bombay (Haffkine Institute in Mumbai is named after him).

Plague Surveillance

Rat fall (sudden death of a large number of rats) in a locality (rural or urban) is a signal for alert. Health personnel in the "at risk" areas must start immediate thorough investigation and advise prophylactic measures for those at risk.

Storage of food grain in rat-proof houses, proper disposal of garbage, removal of wood piles and other possible shelters for rats are helpful as long-term measures of control of plague. Early warning signals include positive serology in rodents, high flea index, evidence of rat fall and suspected human case.

For adequate rodent control, houses and warehouses should be rat-proofed. Rat control on ships and in docks is also very important.

BIBLIOGRAPHY

1. Butler T, Bell WR, Link NN, Tiep ND, Arnold K. *Yersinia pestis* infection in Vietnam - Clinical and haematologic aspects. J Infect Dis 1974;129:S78-S84.
2. Butler T. A clinical study of bubonic plague: observations of the 1970 Vietnam epidemic with emphasis on coagulation studies, skin histology and electrocardiograms. Am J Med 1972;53:L 268-76.
3. Butler T. Plague and other *Yersinia* infections. New York: Plenum press; 1983.
4. Center for disease control and prevention. Fatal human plague in Arizona and Colorado;1996 MMWR 1997;46:617.
5. Dennis DT, Campbell GL. Plague and other *Yersinia* infections. In: Fauci AS, Braunwald E, Kasper DL, et al. (Eds). Harrison's Principles of Internal Medicine 17th edn. Mc Graw Hill, New York;2008.pp.980-7.
6. Hudson BW, Wolff K, Butler T. The use of solid phase radio immunoassay techniques for serodiagnosis of human plague infection. Bull Pan Am Health Organ 1980;14:244 -50.
7. Hull HF, Montes JM, Mann JM. Septicaemic plague in New Mexico. J Infect Dis 1987;155:113-8.
8. Lemaitre BC, Mazigh DA, Seavizzi MR. Failure of beta-lactam antibiotics and marked efficiency of fluoroquinolones in treatment of murine *Yersinia pseudotuberculosis* infection. Antimicrob. Agents Chemother 1991;35:1785-90.

9. Mann JM, Martone WJ, Boyce JM, Kaufmann AF, Barnes AM, Weber NS. Endemic human plague in New Mexico: risk factors associated with infection. J Infect Dis 1979;140:397-401.
10. Marshall JD, Quy DV, Gibson FL. Asymptomatic pharyngeal plague infection in Vietnam. Am J Trop Med Hyg 1967;16:175-7.
11. Plague: Surveillance and control. In: CD Alert (Eds). Agarwal SP, et al. 2002;2: 1-16.
12. Slack P. The black death, past and present 2. Some historical problems. Trans Roy, Soc Trop Med Hyg 1989;3:461-3.
13. Smith MD. Plague. In: Cook GC, Zumla A (Eds). Manson's Tropical Diseases. 22nd edn. Saunders Elsevier London; 2009.pp.1119-25.
14. William JE, Arntzen L, Tyndal OL, Isacson M. Application of enzyme immunoassays for the confirmation of clinically suspect plague in Namibia, 1982. Bull World Health Organ 1986;64:745-52.
15. Winter CC, Moody MD. Rapid identification of *Pasteurella pestis* with fluorescent antibody. II. Specific identification of *Pasteurella pestis* in dried smears. J Infect Dis 1959;104:281-7.

14 Chapter Leptospirosis

TK Dutta, RK Sahoo

INTRODUCTION

Leptospirosis is one of the common zoonoses with world wide distribution. In tropical countries, especially in India, it is one of the most wide-spread infections. It is a widely prevalent infectious disease in southern states of India especially Tamil Nadu, Kerala and Andaman. It is, however, an under-diagnosed, under-reported and neglected disease. It is also associated with several types of occupational and recreational activities, and has a wide spectrum of clinical manifestations—mild leptospiral febrile illness to a full-fledged disease with jaundice, renal dysfunction and hemorrhagic diathesis which is referred to as *Weil's syndrome*. It is often associated with multiorgan failure and fatal outcome.

HISTORY

Leptospirosis is a zoonotic disease caused by pathogenic spirochete of the genus *Leptospira*. Leptospirosis often is referred to as Swineherd's disease, swamp fever or mud fever. In 1907, Stimson described the microorganism in renal tubules of a patient who died of so-called yellow fever. The spirochete was first isolated in Japan by Inada and co-workers in 1916, nearly 30 years after Weil described the clinical disease in 1886. Its relatively recent discovery belies the long history of leptospirosis, which was probably known much earlier in China and Japan by names such as *"rice harvest jaundice" and "autumn fever"*. The genus *Leptospira* contains both pathogenic and nonpathogenic strains.

THE PATHOGEN

The disease is caused by the pathogen leptospires. These are coiled, thin, highly motile organism with hooked end and are 6 to 20 µm long and 0.1 µm wide **(Fig. 14.1)**.

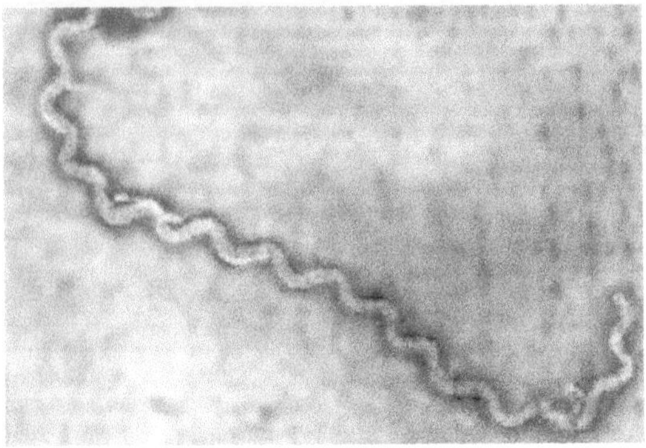

Fig. 14.1: Scanning electron micrograph of *Leptospirae*

SPECIES

Genus *Leptospira* is broadly divided into two species: *Leptospira interrogans* comprising all pathogenic strains and *Leptospira* biflexa, containing the saprophytic (non-pathogenic) strains isolated from the environment. Species *Leptospira interrogans,* comprises of at least 250 antigenically distinct variants knows as serovars belonging to 23 serogroups.

Identification and classification of species of *Leptospira* is important because of different host specialities. This disease has been described as the most common zoonosis affecting many species of wild and domestic animals such as rodents, livestock, wild mammals, dogs and cats. The most frequent hosts are rodents, especially the common rat (*Rattus* norvegicus). In this and other reservoir species, the organisms persist indefinitely in the convoluted tubules of the kidney without causing apparent disease, and are shed in the urine in massive number. Particular serovars are associated with characteristic animal hosts, e.g. *L. icterohaemorrhagiae/copenhageni* is the classical parasite of rats, *L. grippotyphosa* of voles, *L. canicola* of dogs, *L. hardjo* of cattle and *L. pomona* of pigs.

EPIDEMIOLOGY

The disease has worldwide distribution. Human infection can occur either through direct contact with infected animals or much more commonly through indirect contact with water or soil contaminated by urine of infected rodents or animals. Person-to-person transmission is extremely rare since man is the dead-end host for leptospiral dissemination. In contrast, leptospires can survive for long periods in the renal tubules of infected animals without causing illness. Most human infections occur in young adult men and children and result from occupational or environmental exposure. Epidemiological studies indicate that infection is commonly associated with certain occupational workers such as farmer, sewage worker, veterinarian, paddy field worker and animal handler. Leptospirosis can also be transmitted during recreational activities such as hiking, picnicking, swimming, wind surfing, white water rafting and canoeing. Leptospires can survive in untreated water for months or years, but cannot survive desiccation on salt water. The majority of cases occur in the warm season and in rural areas because leptospires can persist in water for many months. They survive best in fresh water, damp alkaline soil, vegetation and mud with temperatures higher than 22°C. Only sporadic cases of leptospirosis are seen in arid climates and deserts. In comparison, the disease is endemic in tropical areas, with heavy precipitation and areas with high levels of subsurface water. Hence, China, Southeast Asia, Africa and South and Central America have immense areas where the disease is endemic. A waterborne outbreak occurred in Italy in the summer of 1984 when a contaminated water fountain was used as a source of drinking water. Leptospirosis occurs sporadically throughout the year in these areas, with a peak seasonal incidence in summer. Large epidemics are reported after monsoons and periods of unusally heavy rainfall. In India, Kerala, Tamil Nadu and Andamans are endemic for leptospirosis. But now with better facilities to detect the disease, the disease is being reported from almost all parts of India.

In a study conducted all over the country by National Reference Center, Regional Medical Research Center (ICMR), Port Blair during the period 2000 to 2001, a seropositivity rate ranging from 0 to 46.8% amongst all cases of fever was observed from various parts of India. The positivity rate was highest in south India at 25.6%. It was 8.3%, 3.5%, 3.1% and 3.3% in northern, western, eastern and central India respectively. Cases of leptospirosis were reported throughout the year in majority of hospitals. 32% of urban slum children in Mumbai had acute leptospirosis during monsoon.

Several outbreaks of leptospirosis have occurred lately. An outbreak emerged in Orissa following supercyclone in 1999.

Transmission via laboratory accidents may occur, but it is rare.

Leptospires from the Greek word leptos, (fine and spiral, a coil) are finely coiled, filamentous spirochetes measuring 6 to 20 mm in length and 0.1 m in width with characteristic curved or hooked ends. Human infection occurs by direct contact with urine or blood of an infected rodent or animal, or from water, soil or vegetable contaminated by urine. The organisms can penetrate abraded skin or intact mucous membrane, after which they enter the circulation and rapidly disseminate to various tissues **(Fig. 14.2)**. There are two distinct phases of leptospiral infection in the body —first, septicemic phase and second, immune phase.

The pathogenesis of leptospirosis is not fully understood **(Fig. 14.3)**. In the septicemic animal models, vascular injury is seen in various organs. Spirochetes can be found in the walls of capillaries and medium—and large sized vessels. The exact mechanism of vascular damage is not clear. A direct

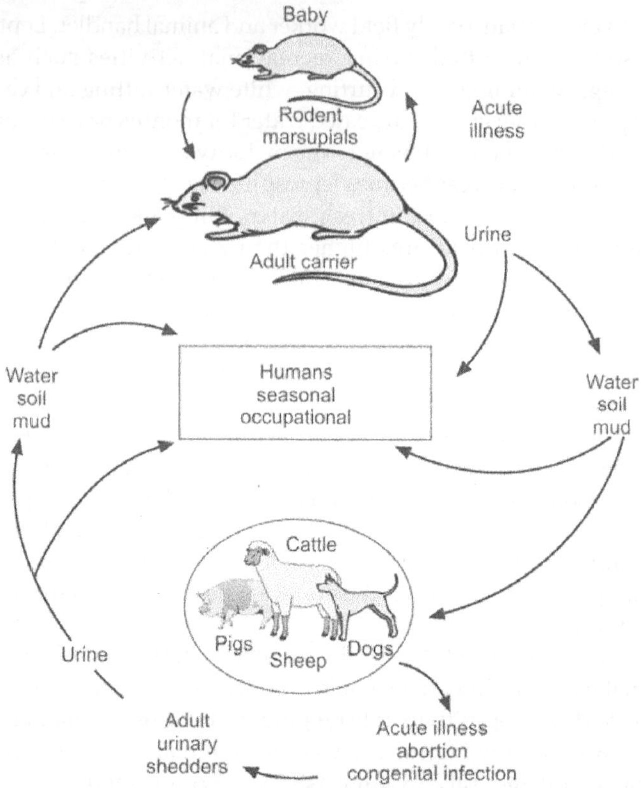

Fig. 14.2: *Leptospira* and leptospirosis

toxic effect of the leptospires has been proposed as cause of the vascular injury, but no bacterial endotoxin has been demonstrated.

In the immune (second) phase of illness, the host immune response, including immune complex deposition may play a role in endothelial injury.

During septicemic phase, invading leptospires are distributed throughout the body. Penetration and invasion of tissues is presumably accomplished through a burrowing motion produced by a pair of axial filaments and release of hyaluronidase. The dissemination and proliferation of spirochetes in various tissues results in a systemic illness, which has a broad spectrum of clinical manifestation. Generalized petechiae and ecchymosis occur in most internal organs in a severe case. Main organs affected are kidney, liver, brain and meninges. Microscopically, a systemic vasculitis with endothelial injury is seen. The damaged endothelial cells usually show different degrees of swelling, necrosis and denudation. The main histopathologic changes are usually found in the liver, kidney, heart and lungs. Hepatic lesions include mild degenerative changes in

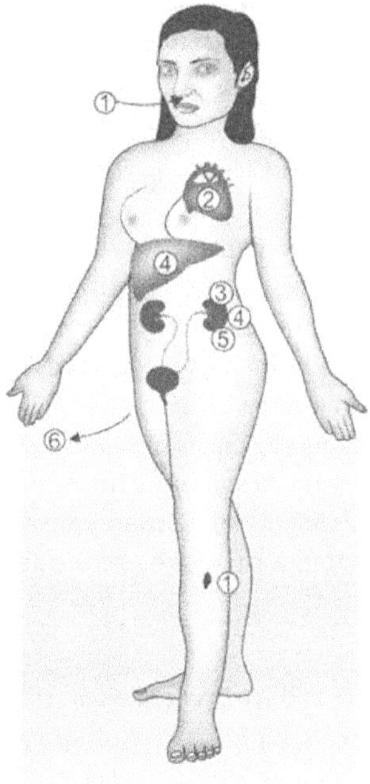

Fig. 14.3: Pathogenesis of leptospirosis

hepatocytes, prominent hypertrophy and hyperplasia of Kupfer cells, erythrophagocytosis and cholestasis. Focal necrosis with occasional acidophilic bodies may occur, but there is no particular zonal distribution associated with the necrosis. Mild to moderate mononuclear cell infiltrates are present in portal tracts. In the kidney, the main histopathologic feature is diffuse tubulointerstitial inflammation characterized by cellular infiltration with lymphocytes, plasma cells, macrophages and polymorphonuclear leukocytes. Tubular necrosis is also a common finding. Glomeruli show mild hyperplasia of mesangial cells and occasional infiltration with inflammatory cells. Grossly the lungs are heavy and severely congested with focal areas of hemorrhage. Microscopically the lungs show congestion with foci of intra-alveolar hemorrhage. In some cases pulmonary lesions include diffuse alveolar damage and variable degrees of airspace disorganization.

1. Water or animal urine contaminated with *Leptospira* sp. splashes onto mucous membrane or abraded skin
2. The bacteria infect the blood stream and are carried throughout all the body tissues causing fever, intense pain
3. Symptoms subside and bacteria disappear from blood and tissues except kidneys

4. Symptoms recur associated with severe damage to liver and kidneys
5. Complete recovery occurs if kidney failure can be effectively treated
6. Excretion of *Leptospira* continues in urine

Leptospires also may invade skeletal muscle, causing edema, vacuolization of myofibrils and focal necrosis. Muscular microcirculation is impaired and capillary permeability is increased with resultant fluid leakage and circulatory hypovolemia.

In severe disease, a disseminated vasculitic syndrome may result from damage to the capillary endothelium. Leptospires may invade the aqueous humor of the eye, where they may persist for many months, occasionally leading to chronic or recurrent uveitis.

Despite the possibility of severe complications, the disease is mostly self-limited and nonfatal. Overtime, a systemic immune response may eliminate the organism from the body, but it also may lead to a symptomatic inflammatory reaction that can produce secondary end-organ injury.

Clinical Manifestations

In its mild form, leptospirosis may present as an influenza—like illness with headache and myalgia. Severe leptospirosis, characterized by jaundice, renal dysfunction, and hemorrhagic diathesis, is referred to as Weil's syndrome.

Incubation Period: 2 to 26 days (usually 7–12 days)

In general, clinical manifestation can be divided into two distinct clinical syndromes. 90% of patients present with mild anicteric febrile illness; 10% are severely ill with jaundice and other manifestations (Weil's disease). Both anicteric and icteric leptospirosis may follow a biphasic course **(Table 14.1)**.

Anicteric leptospirosis is the more common and milder form of the disease and is often biphasic. In the first or septicemic phase, patients usually present with an abrupt onset of fever, chills, headache, myalgia, skin rash, nausea, vomiting, conjunctival suffusion and prostration. Leptospires can be isolated from blood, cerebrospinal fluid (CSF), and tissues. The fever

Table 14.1: Leptospirosis: Anicteric and Icteric

Leptospirosis	*Anicteric*		*Icteric*		
	First stage 3–7 days (Septicemic)	Second stage 0–30 days (Immune)	First stage 3–7 days 3–8 (Septicemic)		Second stage 0–30 days (Immune)
Clinical findings	Fever, myalgia, Headache, conjunctival suffusion, abdominal pain, vomiting	Menigitis uveitis rash, fever		High fever Jaundice Hemorrhages Renal failure	
Leptospires present	Blood CSF	Urine		Blood CSF	Urine

may be high and remittent reaching a peak of 40°C before defervescence. Conjunctival suffusion is characteristic and usually appears on the third or fourth day. Myalgia usually occurs and pain in the muscles in the calf, abdomen and paraspinal region can be severe. When present in the neck, myalgias may cause nuchal rigidity reminiscent of meningitis. In the abdomen, myalgia may mimic acute abdomen, leading to confusion with surgical intra-abdominal emergencies. The skin manifestations seen in mild leptospirosis include transient urticarial, macular or maculopapular, erythematous or purpuric rash. The first phase lasts 3 to 9 days followed by 2 to 3 days of defervescence, after which the second "immune" phase develops.

The immune phase, is characterized by leptospiruria and correlates with the appearance of IgM antibodies in the serum. *Leptospira* now settle in glomeruli and are eliminated from all sites in the host except eye and perhaps brain, where they may persist for weeks or months. Fever and earlier constitutional symptoms recur in some patients, and signs of meningitis, such as headache, photophobia, and nuchal rigidity may develop. Central nervous system (CNS) involvement in leptospirosis most commonly occurs as aseptic meningitis. Complications such as optic neuritis, uveitis, iridocyclitis, chorioretinitis, and peripheral neuropathy occur more frequently in the immune phase. Prolonged or recurrent uveitis was demonstrated in 2% of patients with onset several months after symptoms of clinical leptospirosis. A rare but severe manifestation is hemorrhagic pneumonia. The illness in anicteric leptospirosis may be self-limited, lasting 4 to 30 days, with complete recovery as a rule.

In icteric leptospirosis (Weil's syndrome) usually caused by *L. icterohaemorrhagiae*, persistent high fever and jaundice may obscure the two phases. This is usually associated with hepatic dysfunction, renal insufficiency, hemorrhage and multi-organ failure (MOF). Hemorrhage can occur as petechiae, purpura, conjunctival hemorrhage and gastrointestinal hemorrhage. MOF is associated with a very high mortality. Myocarditis and hemorhagic pulmonary infiltration are other complications, which may prove fatal.

Pulmonary Syndrome

An exclusive pulmonary syndrome has long been recognized in the Far East. The syndrome is characterized by hemoptysis, patchy lung infiltrates on chest X-ray, and respiratory failure. Total bilateral lung consolidation and the ARDS develop in fatal cases. Almost with similar presentation and high mortality, leptospirosis with early pulmonary symptoms including hemoptysis and other hemorrhagic manifestations in Andaman was called as *Andaman hemorrhagic fever*. It was long considered to be a viral hemorrhagic fever, before *Leptospira* as etiological agent was identified in 1993. Severe pulmonary hemorrhage has also been described in China, Korea and Nicaragua, where patients died due to this.

UNCOMMON MANIFESTATIONS

Less common manifestation of leptospirosis is hemorrhage with no significant renal dysfunction or jaundice, when it may be mistaken for dengue hemorrhagic fever. Other uncommon manifestations are generalized lymphadenopathy, pharyngitis and acalculous cholecysitis.

INVESTIGATION

Most of the routine labroratory tests show nonspecific findings. The leukocyte count can be low, normal or elevated, but is usually associated with a shift to left. Mild anemia and thrombocytopenia are common; hemolytic anemia and disseminated intravascular coagulopathy (DIC) have been described in severe cases. Thromobocytopenia is found in more than 50% of patients and is significantly associated with renal failure. Liver, kidney and central nervous system involvement may be present in any combination. Liver involvement may be mild or severe with bilirubin levels reaching very high. Serum alkaline phosphatase, lactate dehydrogenase, aspartate aminotransferase (AST) and alanine aminotransferase (ALT) may all be elevated, but serum AST is only mildly or moderately elevated (unlike in viral hepatitis). Hyperamylasemia occurs frequently in severe disease, but pancreatitis is rare. Serum creatinine phosphokinase (CPK) is usually raised due to muscular involvement.

Proteinuria, pyuria, hematuria, and hyaline or granular casts are common findings on urine analysis even in the absence of renal dysfunction. Renal dysfunction is primarily a result of tubular damage; however, hypovolemia may play a critical role in the subsequent development of renal insufficiency.

In the cerebrospinal fluid (CSF), features are those of aseptic meningitis. The CSF protein level may be normal or elevated upto 300 mg/dl, while the glucose concentration is normal. Although abnormal CSF findings are reported in as many as 80% of leptospirosis cases, only half of the patients are symptomatic.

Various electrocardiographic and chest X-ray abnormalities are observed in patients with leptospirosis. Arrhythmias due to significant cardiac irritability have been documented. The arrhythmias observed were atrial fibrillation, atrial flutter, atrial tachycardia and premature ventricular contractions. Echocardiograms may reveal paricarditis and small pericardial effusions in few cases. The chest radiographic abnormalities can include pulmonary edema, diffuse pneumonitis, nonsegmental or basal linear opacities and pleural effusions.

Diagnosis (Table 14.2)

Definitive diagnosis of leptospirosis depends on:

- Isolation of organism
- Serological tests
- Detection of specific DNA.

Table 14.2: Diagnosis of leptospirosis

Isolation of organism

1. Before tenth day of illness: Blood
   a. Dark field examination of the patient's blood
   b. Culture on a semisolid medium (e.g.Fletcher's EMJH)
2. After tenth day of illness: Urine
   a. Dark field examination of the patient's urine
   b. Culture of urine (for several months in untreated patient)

Serology

Agglutination tests: Paired sera (Fourfold or greater rise in titre)
   a. Microscopic, using live organism (MAT)
   b. Macroscopic, using killed antigen

ELISA IgM and Slide agglutination tests (SAT)
   - Measure IgM antibodies
   - Single sample adequate
   - The ELISA IgM test helpful for early diagnosis (positive 2 days into illness)

Dot-ELISA and dip-stick methods
   - Newer screening methods (for detecting IgM antibodies)

PCR test for Leptospiral DNA
   - Detected in blood, urine, CSF, and aqueous humor

*Specific servoar is detected only by microscopic agglutination test (MAT) and culture isolation

Isolation of Organism

- *Blood:* The organism may be identified by dark field examination of the patient's blood or by culture on a semisolid medium (e.g. Fletcher's EMJH, i.e. Ellinghausen-McCullough -Johnson-Harris), if taken before the tenth day of illness. Cultures take 1 to 6 weeks to become positive.
- *Urine:* The organism may be isolated from the urine on darkground microscopy tenth day onwards, and in untreated patient, may be recovered on urine culture for several months.

Serology

Diagnosis is usually made by means of serologic tests, of which several are available.

- Agglutination tests (microscopic, using live organisms; and macroscopic, using killed antigen) become positive after 7 to 10 days of illness, peak at 3 to 4 weeks, and may persist at high levels for many years. Thus, to make a diagnosis, a fourfold or greater rise in titer must be documented. The agglutination tests are cumbersome to perform and require trained personnel.
- ELISA IgM and slide agglutination tests (SAT) are also available.

As ELISA IgM and slide agglutination tests (SAT) are simple, sensitive tests which measure IgM antibodies, they are used to diagnose current leptospirosis at a very early stage and a single sample is adequate. The IgM

ELISA test is particularly useful in making an early diagnosis, as it is positive as early as 2 days into illness, a time when the clinical manifestation may be nonspecific. It was found to be 100% sensitive and 93% specific in one study. Dot-ELISA and dip-stick methods for detecting IgM antibodies are newer screening methods. Other serological tests available are indirect fluorescent antibody test (IFAT), indirect hemagglutination test (IHAT), latex agglutination test (LAT), micro-capsule agglutination text (MicAT), counter immuno-electrophoresis (CIE) and CFT.

Detection of Specific DNA

Polymerase chain reaction (PCR) methods (presently investigational) appear to be sensitive, specific, positive early in disease, and are able to detect leptospiral DNA in blood, urine, cerebrospinal fluid (CSF) and aqueous humor. Currently major disadvantage with these tests is that these are genus-specific, not serovar specific.

Specific Serovar

The investigation of choice to identity specific serovar is microscopic agglutination test (MAT) and culture isolation. However, culture growth may take several weeks.

WHO GUIDELINES

Faine's criteria for diagnosis of leptospirosis:

Faine had evolved criteria for diagnosis of leptospirosis on the basis of clinical, epidemiological and laboratory data (Parts A, B and C respectively) **(Table 14.3)**.

A presumptive diagnosis of leptospirosis may be made if:

- Parts A and B score=26 or more (Part C laboratory report is usually not available before fifth day of illness; thus it is mainly a clinical and epidemiologic diagnosis during early part of disease)
- Part A+B+C=25 or more

A score between 20 and 25: Suggests a possible but unconfirmed diagnosis of leptospirosis.

Shiva Kumar et al. from Chennai have suggested modification on Faine's criteria to include local factor (like rainfall) and newer investigations in the total scoring. As per this, epidemiological and laboratory criteria (Parts B and C) are modified only; no modification is made in the clinical criteria (Part A) **(Table 14.3)**.

The reasons for modification suggested are as follows:

Most of the leptospirosis is reported in monsoon and post-monsoon period. Therefore, they have suggested rainfall separately to be adjusted in the scoring criteria of Part B.

Microscopic agglutination test (MAT) is the gold standard for diagnosis, but it is complicated and less sensitive compared to newer tests like ELISA IgM and slide agglutination tests. ELISA IgM and slide agglutination tests (SAT) are simple, sensitive tests and can be used to diagnose current leptospirosis. Thus, they have been included with appropriate score.

The difficulties in utilizing MAT are due to the following reasons:

- The antibody titers rise and peak only in second or third week. Thus, paired sera are required to demonstrate 4-fold rise of titer.
- The test is complicated requiring dark-field microscopy and cultures of various serovars, which may not be available in smaller laboratories.

The advantage of including simple diagnostic test is:

ELISA IgM or SAT tests (in modified Faine's criteria) help in diagnosing milder forms of leptospirosis which are associated with low clinical score (Part A).

Table 14.3: Scoring criteria for diagnosis of leptospirosis

Faine's Criteria	*Score*	*Modified Faine's Criteria*	*Score*
Part A:Clinical data			
Headache	2	Headache	2
Fever	2	Fever	2
If fever, temperature 39°C or more	2	If fever, temperature 39°C or more	2
Conjunctival suffusion(Bilateral)	4	Conjunctival suffusion(bilateral)	4
Meningism	4	Meningism	4
Muscle pain(Especially calf muscle)	4	Muscle pain (Especially calf muscle)	4
Conjunctival suffusion+Meningism+ muscle pain	10	Conjunctival suffusion+<eningism+ muscle pain	10
Jaundice	1	Jaundice	1
Albuminuria or nitrogen retention	2	Albuminuria or nitrogen retention	2
Part B: Epidemiological factors			
Contact with animals or contact with known contaminated water	10	Rainfall	5
		Contact with contaminated environment	4
		Animals	1
		Total	10
Part C: Bacteriological and lab findings			
Isolation of leptospirosis in culture – diagnosis certain		Isolation of leptospirosis in culture – diagnosis certain	
Positive serology (MAT)		**Positive serology**	
Leptospirosis endemic:			
Single positive low titer	2	ELISA IgM positive*	15
Single positive high titer	10	SAT positive*	15
Leptaspirosis nonendemic:			
Single positive low titer	5	MAT single high titer*	15
Single positive high titer	15	MAT rising titer (Paired sera)	25
Rising titer (paired sera)	25		
Total score		Total score	

* Any one of the tests only should be scored

Suggestion for modification of existing Faine's criteria appears justified; however, further evaluation is required.

DIFFERENTIAL DIAGNOSIS

The differential diagnosis of leptospirosis depends on the epidemiology of acute febrile illnesses in the particular area. A high index of suspicion is needed in endemic areas, and leptospirosis must be considered when a patient presents with acute onset of fever, headache and myalgia. However, in locations where dengue fever or malaria is also present, the differentiation may be very difficult because of similar clinical manifestations. Laboratory confirmation is crucial, especially when these diseases are occurring simultaneously during the rainy season. Other conditions to be considered in the differential diagnosis include influenza, meningitis (or encephalitis), viral hepatitis, rickettsiosis, typhoid fever, septicemia, toxoplasmosis and Legionnaire's disease.

When the patient presents with jaundice during or after an acute febrile illness, leptospirosis must be differentiated from other causes of febrile jaundice such as malaria, septicemia, alcoholic hepatitis and typhoid hepatitis.

The high bilirubin level seen in Weil's disease with mild to modest elevation of transaminases assists in differentiating it from viral hepatitis where there is usually a much higher elevation of transaminases. Further, a high serum creatinine phosphokinase (CPK) concentration or thrombocytopenia also favors a diagnosis of leptospirosis. Serum CPK is usually found normal in viral hepatitis.

TREATMENT

Various antimicrobial drugs, including penicillin and tetracyclines, show antileptospiral activity **(Table 14.4)**. Penicillin (e.g. 6 million units daily) and ceftriaxone (e.g. 2 gm daily) are the drugs of choice in severe leptospirosis and are especially effective if started within first four days of illness. Total duration of therapy should be 10 to 14 days.

Table 14.4: Drug treatment and prophylaxis of leptospirosis*

	Drug	*Route*	*Dose*
	Doxycycline	Oral	100 mg bid
Mild leptospirosis	Ampicillin	Oral	500–700 mg qid
	Amoxycillin	Oral	500 mg qid
Moderate/severe leptospirosis	Penicillin G	IV	1.0–1.5 millon unit qid
	Ceftriaxone	IV	1–2 gm od
	Ampicillin	IV	1 gm qid
	Erythromycin	IV	500 mg qid
Prophylaxis	Doxycycline	Oral	200 mg once aweek

*In all regimens, drugs used for treatment are administered for 7 days

Amoxycillin and erythromycin have also been found effective in severe leptospirosis. Patient should be observed for evidence of renal failure, and treated, if necessary, with hemodialysis. Patients with Weil's disease having hemorrhagic manifestation may require whole blood or platelet transfusion. Patients with multi-organ failure require to be observed in intensive care unit.

Besides penicillin, doxycycline in a dosage of 100 mg twice daily for 7 days is effective in mild and moderate leptospirosis.

Effective prophylaxis consists of doxycycline, 200 mg orally once weekly, during the exposure.

PROGNOSIS

The prognosis of leptospirosis depends on the severity of the disease and associated complications. Pregnant women also face a high-rate of fetal mortality, as infected women have higher than normal incidence of spontaneous abortion if the infection is acquired in the early months of pregnancy. Patients with hepatic dysfunction and renal failure have a good chance of recovery in long-term. Anicteric leptospirosis usually has a good prognosis. Without jaundice the disease is almost never fatal; however, fatal pulmonary hemorrhage and myocarditis have been reported occasionally in anicteric cases. The case fatality rate for Weil's disease is 15 to 40% and is higher for patients over 60 years of age.

PREVENTION

Following measures can be adopted to prevent leptospirosis. Protective clothings should be worn by those exposed to contaminated water or soil because of their job or recreational activities. Personal protective equipment while handling infected animal or tissue includes gloves, face shields for veterinarians and rubber boots for sewer worker and agriculture worker who work in rodent urine contaminated water. Vaccines are offered to high-risk workers in some European and Asian countries (e.g. rice worker in Italy). Human vaccines are serovar specific and must be repeated yearly. Immunizing and treating infected animals is worthwhile. Animal vaccines are also serovar specific.

Hence the vaccine given should contain the serovars known to be prevalent in that area. Chemo-prophylaxis with doxycycline (200 mg twice a week) is effective during the risk of exposure.

SUMMARY

- Leptospirosis is a zoonotic disease caused by pathogenic spirochetes belonging to the genus *Leptospira* and occurs in endemic and epidemic forms in many parts of the world as in India.
- Human infection occurs by direct contact with urine or blood of an infected rodent or animal, or water, soil or vegetable contaminated by urine.

- The incubation period is usually 7 to 12 days, with a range of 2 to 26 days.
- Ninety percent patients present with anicteric febrile illness. Ten percent patients present with severe illness, jaundice and other manifestations like myositis and conjunctivitis. Hepatic and renal involvement and hemorrhagic diathesis are referred to as Weil's syndrome.
- Definitive diagnosis of leptospirosis depends on - isolation of organism, serological test and detection of specific DNA.
- IgM ELISA, Dot-ELISA, dip-stick method and slide agglutination test (SAT) are earliest to be positive (IgM ELISA 2nd day into illness), thus are good screening test, however reports are not genus specific.
- Identifying specific serovar is possible by Microscopic agglutination test (MAT) and culture method only.
- Faine's criteria for diagnosis of leptospirosis may be made, if part A + B scores>=26 or part A + B + C score>=25 as per **(Table 14.3)**.
- Anicteric type of disease is easily treatable with penicillin and/or doxycyline and has good prognosis.
- However, patient with renal failure, hemorrhagic diathesis or multi-organ failure may require hemodialysis, whole blood or platelet transfusion or need to be observed in intensive care unit.
- Oral doxycyline can be used for prophylaxis during the risk of exposure.

BIBLIOGRAPHY

1. Agrawal A, Biswajit D, Rajan SK, Dutta TK, Kumar K, Mathai D. Infectious disease. Medicine Update: The Association of Physicians of India 2003;13:73-6.
2. Christopher AM, Mohapatra AK, Binay, Dutta TK, Kanungo R, Das AK. Pulmonary manifestations of leptospirosis. In: Souvenir, 3rd Annual Conference of Indian Leptospirosis Society, Pondicherry 2002.p.32.
3. Dutta TK, Christopher M. Leptospitosis. An Overview. J Assoc Physic India 2005;53:545-50.
4. Faine S. Guidelines for the control of leptospirosis. WHO Offset Publication No. 67, Geneva 1982.
5. Kamath S. Leptospirosis In: Das S (Ed). API Medicine Update, Mumbai 2003; 13:1008-11.
6. Kamath SA, Joshi SR. Re-emerging infections in urban India - Focus Leptospirosis. J Assoc Physic India 2003;51:247-8.
7. Philip SS, Jacobs RA. Spirochetal infections In: Mc Phee SJ, Papadakis MA (Eds). Current medical Diagnosis and Treatment. 48th edn. Mc Graw Hill, New York 2009.pp.1297-1304.
8. Sehgal SC. Leptospirosis - an unresolved enigma of the twentieth century. In: Souvenir, 1st National Leptospirosis Conference, Bangalore 1999.pp.16-20.
9. Shiva Kumar S, Shareek PS. Diagnosis of leptospirosis utilizing modified Faine's criteria. J Assoc Physic India 2004;52:678-9.
10. Speelman P, Hartskeerl R. Leptospirosis. In: Fauci AS, Braunwald E, Kasper DL, et al. (Eds). Harrison's Principles of Internal Medicine 17th edn. Mc Graw Hill, New York 2008.pp.1048-51.
11. Weil A. Ueber eine eigentimiliche, mitMilztumor, Icterus, and Nephritis einhergehends acute Infektionskrankheti. Dtsch Arch Klin Med 1886;39:209.

15 Yaws: A Global Menace

Chapter

JK Dutta

With ardent efforts by World Health Organization (WHO), small pox has been eradicated from the globe. Several other communicable diseases like rabies, malaria, tuberculosis, plague, leprosy, AIDS also need to be eradicated from tropical countries where they claim heavy toll of life every year. Yaws, a disease common among the unprivileged tribals also needs eradication at the earliest.

Global Scenario

Yaws even now is prevalent in Africa, Central and South America, the Caribbean, South-East-Asia including in India. Previously it was endemic in several countries like Germany, Spain, Portugal, France, etc.

In local language the disease is known as *Frambesia* (German), Buba (Spanish), Bouba (Portuguese), Pian (French), Coko (Fiji), Bubas (Brazil). In 1952–1964, WHO in collaboration with UNICEF launched the global endemic treponematoses control program as a result of which more than 50 million patients in 46 countries were treated and the incidence was drastically reduced though not totally eradicated.

Since 1970 onwards there has been resurgence of the disease in many regions in the world. In 1980's and 1990's resurgence occurred in West and Central Africa, South Pacific regions and some South-East Asian countries. The inhabitants still continue to be victims of this scourge.

Indian Scenario

Yaws was first recognized among laborers working in tea plantations in Assam in 1887. In India the disease is known in different names in different areas like "*Media Roga*" in Chattisgarh, "*Goudi Roga*" in Maharashtra, "*Koya Rogam*" in Andhra Pradesh, "Domaru Khahu" in Assam, "Chakwar" in Uttar Pradesh.

After a sharp decline as a result of mass campaign by WHO and UNICEF in 1950, there has been a resurgence of the disease in India. Currently the disease is prevalent mostly among tribal population living in hilly and forest areas of Orissa, Andhra Pradesh, Chattisgarh, Madhya Pradesh, Tamil Nadu, Assam, Bihar, Uttar Pradesh and Gujarat.

Etiology

Yaws is caused by *Treponema pallidum* subspecies *pertinue*. Two other similar microbes, *Treponema pallidum* subspecies *endemicum* causes endemic syphilis (bijel) and *T. pallidum* subspecies *carateum* causes pinta.

The causative agent of yaws is morphologically and immunologically similar to *Treponema pallidum* which causes venereal syphilis. It is a spiral organism visible in dark-field illumination by light microscopy. It cannot be grown in artificial media.

Epidemiology

Man is the sole reservoir of infection. The infection usually spreads from cases of early yaws which are infectious. It mainly spreads by person-to-person contact with exudates or discharges from skin lesions of patients. Treponemes can hardly penetrate through intact skin. They usually enter through minor skin lesion or abrasion. Transmission of infection usually increases in rainy season. Early yaws is primarily observed in children and adolescents.

Clinical Manifestations

Incubation period of the disease is usually 9 to 90 days. The initial lesion (Mother Yaws) appears at the site of inoculation of the organism. The disease manifests in two phases—early or infectious yaws and late yaws.

Early Yaws

In this phase exudates are noticed on the skin, which dry up to form scabs and yellow crusted granulomatous eruptions. There may be papillomatous eruptions with 'Cauliflower' like appearance of ulcerated papilloma. Regional lymphadenopathy is common. In some patients there may be hyperkeratosis in palms and soles or inflammation of the interphalangeal joints (polydactylitis) or periosteitis of long bone causing nocturnal pain. Papillomatous eruptions on plantar surface causes limping gait due to pain which is called 'Crab Yaws' as the patient moves like a crab. Hypertrophic osteitis of nasal process of maxilla causes swelling on both sides of the bridge of the nose which is called "Goundou". The lesions in early yaws persist for 3 to 6 months and then heal spontaneously.

Late Yaws

There are destructive and often deforming lesions in this phase which appear after five years or longer. There is gumma formation in skin and subcutaneous tissues. Disfiguring lesions of the nasopharynx result in "Gangosa". Ulceration of the palate may result in perforation of cheek with destruction of the turbinate bone and foul smelling discharge. Goundou and hyperkeratosis of palms and soles are much more pronounced in this stage with deep fissuring. Hypertrophic osteoperiosteitis results in *"Sabre Tibia"* due to which there is pain over the shaft of the tibia particularly at night. Pathological fractures and malunion may result in deformities of the limbs. Usually there is no congenital transmission. Neither the central nervous system nor cardiovascular system is involved. However, involvement of above noted systems has been reported by some investigators lately.

A latent stage is commonly observed in this disease. After initial stage, yaws may remain latent for several months or years. Most of the latent cases are found in clusters around an infectious case.

Histopathological Changes

Histopathological examination of biopsy specimen shows less marked endothelial proliferation but acanthosis is more prominent. Treponemes may be detected in biopsy specimens collected from cases of early yaws if the specimen is stained by a silver impregnation technique. Paucity of T and B lymphocytes in specimens from yaws cases has been observed by monoclonal antibody technique.

Diagnosis and Differential Diagnosis

In endemic areas diagnosis of yaws is easy clinically when there are characteristic lesions. On dark-field examination of exudates from early lesion, treponemes can be easily identified. Bony lesions like periosteitis, bony hypertrophy can be detected by radiological examination. A number of conditions like endemic syphilis, leprosy, tuberculous skin lesions, fungal infections and psoriasis need to be differentiated from yaws.

Serological Tests

Few serological tests like venereal disease research laboratory (VDRL), rapid plasma reagin (RPR), treponema pallidum hemagglutination (TPHA) and fluorescent treponemal antibody (FTA) are available for diagnosis of treponemal infection.

Treponemal tests are more specific than reagin test. However, they remain positive for life and cannot distinguish between current and past infection. RPR and TPHA are simple to perform. Reagin tests show a falling titre after successful treatment and hence are useful to monitor the efficacy of the treatment.

Treatment

The author had the opportunity to treat several cases of yaws among the tribal population called *"Kandha"* in Ganjam district of Orissa in India in 1940s. During those days of preantibiotic era, arsenic was the drug of choice. Nov arseno billon (NAB) was used in initial dose of 0.15 gm intravenously, and then increased by 0.15 gm every 2 to 3 days to a maximum of 0.60 gm. In total six doses had to be administered in a course. Skin lesions would disappear after 2 to 3 doses. However, completion of the course was essential to prevent relapse. Care had to be taken to inject the drug slowly and carefully into the vein as extravasation of the drug would result in local pain and swelling.

Currently, *Benzathine penicillin* is the drug of choice. For children below 10 years of age 0.6 million units should be injected intramuscularly in a single dose. Double this dose, i.e. 1.2 million units should be used in single dose for those above this age group and 2.4 million units for adults is recommended. Sensitivity to penicillin should be tested by a small dose before using the full dose of the drug. Failure of penicillin therapy is a rare phenomenon.

Alternative drugs may be used for those sensitive to penicillin. These include tetracycline or erythromycin. For children below eight years of age, erythromycin 30 mg/kg should be administered orally in four divided doses daily for 15 days. For those between 8 to 15 years of age, tetracycline or erythromycin 250 mg qid orally and for patients above 15 years, 500 mg of the same drugs may be used by the same route for a period of 15 days. Tetracycline should not be administered to pregnant and lactating women and children below eight years of age.

Yaws Eradication Program

Diagnosis and treatment of the disease is simple. The WHO expert committee on venereal infection and treponematoses have stressed that eradication of yaws is possible from technical point of view. Yaws eradication program was started as a pilot project by Government of India in Koraput district of Orissa during the year 1996 to 1997. The program now covers 49 districts in 10 states of India where the disease is prevalent.

A task force has been formed under the chairmanship of Director General of Health Services, Government of India. Education of the community is an essential component of the program. All important agencies like union ministry of tribal affairs, Integrated Tribal Development Agency (ITDA), state and district health officers, Department of Health and Family Welfare of Government of India, NGO's have been included in the program.

Though success has been achieved in some regions by 2001, the disease is still persisting in several areas. Hence, there is need to continue the program further to achieve the goal of "Total Eradication". A global eradication program is also the need of the hour.

BIBLIOGRAPHY

1. Backhouse JL. Failure of penicillin treatment of yaws on Karkar Island, Papua New Guinea. Am J Trop Med 1998;59:388.
2. Endemic treponematoses in the 1980's Editorial. Lancet 1983;II:551-2.
3. Engelken HJH. Endemic treponematosis. Part 1. Yaws Int J Dermatol 1991; 30:77.
4. Engelkens HJH, Tenkate FJW, Judanarso J, et al. The localization of treponemes and characterization of the inflammatory infiltrate in skin biopsies from patients with primary or secondary syphilis or early infectious yaws. Genitourin Med 1993;69:102-7.
5. Engelkens HJH, Vuzevski VD, Judanarso J, et al. Early Yaws: a light microscopy study. Genitourin Med 1990;66:264-6.
6. Haackett CJ, Loewenthal LJA. The differential Diagnosis of Yaws. Monograph NO. 36. Geneva, World Health Organization 1960.
7. Noordhoek GT, Engelkens HJ, Judanarso J, et al. Yaws in West Sumatra, Indonesia: clinical manifestation, serological finding and characterization of new treponema isolates by DNA probes. Europ J Clin Microb and Infect Dis 1991;10:12-9.
8. Perine PL, Hopkins DR, Niemel PLA, St John RK, Causse G, Antal GM. Handbook of endemic treponematoses: Yaws, Endemic Syphilis and Pinta, Geneva, World Health Organization 1984.
9. Roman GC, Roman LN. Occurrence of congenital, cardiovascular, visceral, neurologic and neuro-ophthalmologic complications of late yaws: a theme for future research. Rev Infect Dis 1986;8:760-70.
10. Smith JL, David NJ, Indgin S, et al. Neuro-ophthalmological study of late yaws and pinta. II. The Caracas project. Br J Vener Dis 1971;47:226-51.
11. World Health Organization. Treponemal infection. Technical Report Series 674. Geneva 1982.pp.16-20.
12. Yaws again. Editorial. Br Med J 1980:1090.

16 Chapter Chikungunya Fever

JK Dutta

Chikungunya is a rare form of viral fever caused by an alpha virus. The name is derived from a "Swahili" word which means to bend-up. Bending or stooped posture develops as a result of arthritis associated with the disease.

Chikungunya virus was first isolated in 1953 from the serum of a febrile patient in Tanganyika (Tanzania). Numerous well documented outbreaks have been reported since then in Africa and South-East-Asia. There is a forest cycle involving monkeys (vervets and baboons) transmitted by Aedes Africanus and other mosquitoes.

Etiology

Chikungunya virus is a member of the family, Togaviridae; Genus alphavirus. The other togaviruses of alphavirus genus include Ross fever, Onyoung-Onyoung, etc. The vector is Aedes egypti mosquito.

Epidemiological Features–Asia

The virus was isolated in Bangkok, Thailand in 1958. Outbreaks of the disease have been reported in Cambodia, Vietnam and Myanmar. Sri Lanka, Indonesia, Phillipines and India have also experienced outbreaks. In 1962, nearly 40,000 patients were treated in Bangkok. Chikungunya nearly disappeared from the area since 1970s. The antibodies to chikungunya virus were rare in children in Bangkok born after 1976. Occasional outbreaks have been reported since 1988 but there has been no severe epidemic.

INDIA

In 1963, there was an outbreak of viral hemorrhagic fever in Calcutta. Chikungunya virus was isolated from some of these cases of viral fever with hemorrhagic manifestations. The outbreak continued from July till December but declined with the end of monsoon rains.

According to the statistics available from hospital records there may have been about 200 deaths during the epidemic within the area of corporation of Calcutta and lakhs of people were infected. Diagnosis was confirmed as chikungunya virus by "Quick CF" test in 35 cases by isolation of virus by intracerebral inoculation of suckling mice.

In 1964, there was an epidemic in south India (Vellore, Madras and Pondicherry). During the period 1965 to 1972 there was decline in the infection. In 1973, a small outbreak was reported from Barsi, in Sholapur district of Maharashtra. There was no outbreak in India from 1973 till 2005.

Re-emergence of Chikungunya Infection-global Scenario

In 1999, there was an outbreak in Port Klang in Malaysia in which 27 persons were affected. In La Reunion 3115 cases of chikungunya infections were notified during the period 27 February, 2005 to 28 March, 2006. Since January 2006 cases have been reported from several countries in South-West Indian ocean like Mayotee, Mauritius (Africa) and Seychelles (Africa). Some imported cases have been reported from France, Germany, Italy, Norway and Switzerland.

Incidence of Re-emerging Infection in India

An outbreak of Chikungunya infection has been reported since December 2005 in different parts of Andhra Pradesh. Out of 386 serum samples collected from these areas 139 were positive for IgM antibodies by MAC ELISA to chikungunya virus which were tested in National Institute of Virology, Pune. There have been large outbreaks in Southern India like Gullaya, Tumkur, Bidar, Raichur, Bellary, Chitradurga, Kolapur and Bijapur districts. In March 2006, there was outbreak in Malegaon in Nasik district and Orissa. In May-June 2006 an outbreak was reported in Salem and Chennai.

Since December 2005, there was outbreak of fever cases in Maharashtra. 34,725 cases of fever were reported from December 2005 till April 5 2006. Blood samples numbering 68 were collected from Malegaon, Nasik, Beed and Latur districts out of which 13 showed high titers of antibody against chikungunya and three were positive for IgM antibody against Dengue virus.

Fever with arthritis was reported in 18,529 cases from Gulbarga, Bidar, Bellary, Raichur, Tumkur, Koppal and Chitradurga districts of Karnataka since 2005. Out of 76 serum samples tested from Bidar, 43 were positive for IgM antibodies against chikungunya virus at National Institute of Virology, Pune.

Clinical Features

The incubation period is 1 to 12 days. In above-noted areas patients developed moderate to high fever, joint pain (mostly small joints), lymphadenopathy and rash as the predominant clinical features. All ages and both sexes were affected although there was preponderance above 15 years of age. The water supply through pipe was only for half an hour a day. So people collected and stored water in plastic or metal containers where potential breeding places were provided for Aedes egypti.

Fever recurs after a break of 1 to 2 days. Bleeding from the gums was complained by many patients. Most patients recover fully over a few weeks and death is rarely reported. A few patients (5–10%) have chronic joint pain with stiffness for years. Enythrocyte sedimentation rate is mildly raised. The joint pain, myalgia, conjunctivitis and maculopapular rash are the features which distinguish the illness from dengue.

Laboratory Diagnosis

It is important to note that specimens should be sent to the laboratory at 2° to 8°C as soon as possible. Do not freeze the whole blood as hemolysis may interfere with the results. If a delay of more than 24 hours is likely for submission, the serum should be separated and stored in a frozen condition. The virus can be isolated within 3 to 4 days of illness.

Serological tests are important for diagnosis. Virus specific lgM antibodies can be detected by capture ELISA which may persist beyond six months. Hemagglutination inhibition (HI) antibodies became positive by 5 to 7 days of illness. Paired sera can be tested for He and N antibodies. It is worth noting that there is cross reaction with other alphaviruses.

Blood for isolation of virus and for detection of virus nucleic acid in sera by RT-PCR should be collected within first five days of illness. The samples should be transported within 48 hours to the referral laboratory in cold preferably frozen state.

Treatment

There is no specific treatment yet available. So, symptomatic measures should be adopted for alleviation of symptoms particularly joint pains. Aspirin should be avoided, but ibuprofen, naproxen or paracetamol may be used.

Control and Prevention

No vaccine is yet available for prevention of this infection. So control of vectors and elimination of breeding sites are the important and effective control measures. For control of mosquito breeding several measures have to be adopted. All water containers like tanks, cisterns, barrels should be tightly covered with lid. Containers where water may collect like old tyres, tin cans, buckets, drums and empty bottles should be removed. Water in bowls for pets should be emptied daily. Larvivorous fish like gambusia, guppy should be introduced in contaminated water tanks that can eat and destroy the mosquito larvae. Tall grass should be cut short.

To avoid mosquito bites mosquito nets treated with insecticides should be used even in day time in endemic areas. Insecticide spray with 2% pyrethrum space spray should be carried out to kill the mosquitoes in highly infested areas. Community participation is essential for effective control of the infection. People should be educated to use personal protective measures like using full sleeve clothes and use of mosquito nets.

They should be encouraged to cooperate in measures necessary for elimination of breeding places of mosquitoes. Mass media should be involved by publications in local news papers, magazine, radio, TV, hoardings, posters, pamphlets and hand bills. Members of medical association, Non-Governmental Organization (NGO) should be actively associated for success of the control programs.

Chikungunya Infection in Pregnancy

Mother to fetus infection occurs between 3 and 4½ months of pregnancy but not before or after that period. There is 48 percent risk of infection at birth if virus is present in mother's blood. Usually more than 90 percent of all infected newborns recover quickly without any sequelae.

BIBLIOGRAPHY

1. Brighton AW, Prozesky OW, De La Harpe A. Chikungunya virus infection. A retrospective study of 107 cases. S Afr Med J 1983;63:313-5.
2. Calisher CH. Alphavirus infections (family Togaviridae). In: Porterfield JS (Ed). Kass Hand book of Infectious Diseases. Exotic viral Infections. London Chapman and Hall 1995.pp.1-18.
3. CD Alert. Chikungunya Fever 2006;10(2):1-8.
4. Center for disease control and prevention. Management of patients with suspected viral haemorrhagic fever. MMWR 1988;37(S-3):1.
5. Johnston RE, Peters CJ. Alphaviruses. In: Fields BN, Knipe DM, Howley PM (Eds). Field's virology. 3rd edn. Philadelphia: Lippincott-Raven; 1996;(1): 843-98.

17 Avian Influenza (Bird Flu)

Chapter

JK Dutta

Avian influenza (bird flu) was first recognized in Italy about 100 years ago. It was then known as "Fowl Plague". The virus usually infects birds less commonly pigs. Although all birds are susceptible to infection, domestic chicken flocks are especially vulnerable.

Avian influenza in birds due to H5N1 has been reported from several Asian countries in recent years. Poultry deaths have been reported in Taiwan caused by H5N2 and in Pakistan by H7 strain. Till December 2005, total number of deaths due to laboratory confirmed infection with H5N1 has been reported to be 69 among 134 infected persons. Out of them highest number of deaths, 42 was from Vietnam followed by 13 deaths from Thailand. In the Editorial in the Lancet (2005 Vol 366) avian influenza has been described as a double edged weapon. If it infects human there may be heavy loss of life. Even if it does not spread to human population, the panic caused by the fear of an impending outbreak is equally damaging.

A 3-year-old boy suffered from an influenza-like illness in May 1997 in Hongkong. He died 12 days later with complications consistent with Reye's syndrome. On laboratory investigation a virus was isolated in cell culture which was identified as influenza type A virus but further characterization was not possible then.

By August same year further investigations with serological and molecular techniques in the Netherlands and USA confirmed that the isolate was A/Hongkong 156/97 (H5N1) which was very closely related to isolate A/Chicken/Hongkong/258/7 (H5N1).

The latter virus was considered representative/equivalent of those responsible for severe outbreaks of disease in three rural chicken farms in Hongkong during March 1997 when several thousand chickens died. On further investigation by molecular analysis the viral hemagglutinins showed a proteolytic cleavage site of the type found in highly pathogenic avian influenza viruses.

By late December 1997 the total number of new cases in human reached the figure of 17. Five out of them died. Persons who had been near live chickens in market places were mostly affected which suggested transmission of virus from chicken to man.

The veterinary authorities slaughtered about 1.1 million chickens in the wholesale market and those with vendors within Hongkong and import of chickens from neighboring areas was stopped. As a result no more cases were detected. Public health authorities thought that human strain might co-circulate with avian influenza virus to generate human and avian reassortant viruses with capacity for direct person-to-person transmission. However, this has not been documented so far. The following year 1998 another avian influenza virus (H9N2) was isolated from two patients suffering from mild influenza in children.

Virus

Avian influenza virus is an influenza A virus of the family orthomyxoviridae. There are two forms of the disease caused by the virus (a) mild form (b) highly pathogenic form (highly pathogenic avian influenza (HPA).

There are three types of avian influenza viruses (ABC) out of which A and B cause human disease. Type A is further subdivided according to the type of protein (H) and (N) on its outer layer. There are 16 H types and 9 N types. H5N1 mutates rapidly and causes disease in man. The current outbreak is caused by H5N1 subtype of influenza A virus.

Character

The virus is killed at 56°C in 2 hours. Deep freezing and boiling kills the virus. It is sensitive to detergents and alcohol. It is difficult to inactivate the virus if encrusted in feces or soil. Bird-flu does not spread by air instead by saliva, nasal secretions and excreta. It affects mostly chickens among the birds. Ducks, cranes and pigs harbor the virus as carrier.

Current Outbreak

The current outbreak of avian influenza which started in Hongkong in 1997 has spread to several countries in the globe. A woman died on February 9, 2006 in Indonesia which put the total figure of deaths from that country as 17. In Germany tests carried out on dead swans showed that they were carrying degenerated bird flu virus. The strain of virus found in dead swans is highly pathogenic and potentially dangerous for human. In Vietnam virus H5N1 was identified in some patients. Tests on dead swans in Italy and Greece have confirmed the presence of H5N1 virus. H5N1 infection has swept South-East-Asia, China, Mongolia, Siberia, Greece, Turkey, Romania, Croatia, Ukraine and many other countries. In India H5N1 has been identified in chickens in Nan durbar district of Maharashtra as well as in some parts of Gujarat.

Clinical Manifestations

Bird

The range of symptoms in birds varies depending on the strain of the virus and its virulence. In some birds there may be no symptom or mild illness with ruffled feathers, droopiness, sudden drop in egg production and diarrhea. In few others the symptoms include incoordination, inability to stand or walk, pin-point hemorrhage, respiratory distress followed by death.

Man

There may be typical influenza like illness with fever, sore throat, cough and myalgia. Acute respiratory distress may be followed by death.

DRUGS

Only two drugs have been found to be effective. Zanamivir (Relenza) and Oseltamivir (Tamiflu) are available for human use. These drugs are neuraminidase inhibitors which block the virus replication. Of late, resistance of virus to Tamiflu has been reported in Japan; 16 to 18% of children treated with the drug developed resistance. Resistance was probably due to mutation in the virus.

Recent studies have shown that both A and B influenza viruses can develop resistance to Zanamivir and Oseltamivir. The virus is also resistant to amantidine and rimantidine.

Zanamivir (Relenza)

It is recommended for use in persons over seven years of age with uncomplicated influenza who have symptoms for less than two days. The recommended dosage is two inhalations daily for five days. Contraindications include asthma and chronic obstructive pulmonary disease.

Oseltamivir (Tamiflu)

The drug is approved for treatment of uncomplicated influenza in individuals over one year of age who have symptoms for less than two days. The recommended dose is 75 mg twice daily orally for five days for adults. For children, the dose is calculated on the basis of weight. This drug is also approved for prevention of influenza A and B in individuals over one year of age. None of these drugs are recommended for use during pregnancy and nursing.

Preventive Measures

Avian Influenza Vaccine for Poultry

Inactivated-whole-virus vaccine is used by subcutaneous or intramuscular administration. The vaccine is produced by using unpurified allantoic fluid emulsified in an oil based proprietary adjuvant.

Avian Influenza Vaccine for Human

Although clinical trials began in 2005, there are no vaccines commercially available yet for humans against H5N1. However some organizations are actively involved in developing a suitable vaccine in future (Sanofi Pasteur and Chiron). Several prototypes are being explored for manufacture of a suitable vaccine for human use.

For prevention of spread of infection, the chickens in affected farms must be culled.

BIBLIOGRAPHY

1. CD Alert. National Institute of Communicable Diseases, Delhi 2005;9:1-8.
2. Clem A, Galwankar S. Avian Influenza: Preparing for a pandemic. J Assoc Physicians Ind 2006;54:563-70.
3. No human case of Avian Influenza reported. Health Ministry, February 24, 2006. www. Webindia 123.com.
4. Shetty NP, Shetty PS. Epidemiology of disease in the tropics. Manson's Tropical Diseases. Cook GC, Zumla A, Saunders Elsevier (Eds). London 22nd edn. 2009.pp.19-34.
5. The Editorial. The Lancet Infectious Disease 2005;366:1751.

18 Chapter

Hantavirus Pulmonary Syndrome

JK Dutta

Whether Hantavirus is an emerging infection is an intriguing question. Clearly it is a newly recognized disease. Sin nimbre virus (SNV) and other American Hantaviruses are newly recognized pathogens like legionella, bartonella, ehrlichia, etc. Based on genetic evidence it is suggested that SNV is not the result of recent genetic mutation but a virus that has coevolved with its rodent host over many years.

History

In 1993, a young healthy man died shortly after collapsing at the funeral of his fiancée in New Mexico. Soon some more deaths were reported resulting mostly from acute respiratory distress syndrome. Finally, a breakthrough was obtained after intense investigation and the causative agent was identified as Hantavirus which was found in Eurasia.

It is named after the Hantan river in South Korea where the prototype virus was first isolated in 1976. The genus "Hantavirus" has at least 30 members which are found worldwide. This virus belongs to family Bunyaviridae. Each Hantavirus has one primary rodent reservoir.

By April 2001, Hantavirus pulmonary syndrome (HPS) cases numbering 283 had been recorded in USA. Nearly 60% of cases were observed in males. Mean age was 37 year (range 10–70 years). More cases were observed in adults compared to children. The case fatality rate in adult is 41%. Deer mouse is the reservoir for SNV in Western United States.

Clinical Features

Hantavirus pulmonary syndrome (HPS) is observed most often in the spring and summer. Incubation period is likely to be between five days and four weeks. In the prodromal phase there is influenza like illness with fever, chill, malaise, myalgia, nausea, vomiting and cough. Thrombocytopenia is usually present at this stage.

Later a shock stage (cardiopulmonary phase) begins which lasts for several days. There is shortness of breath with tachypnea and tachycardia.

In the final stage (convalescent stage) cardiac parameters return to normal but in some patients there may be renal impairment. Usually sore throat and rhinorrhea are absent.

Treatment

No specific treatment is yet available. Hence, supportive measures are of prime importance. Antiviral drugs have a minor role. Shock and hypoxia should be adequately treated. Treatment in a critical care unit is advisable. Mechanical ventilation should be provided by intubation. In Central and South America, patients usually develop hemorrhagic manifestations and proteinuria or hematuria.

Diagnosis

Diagnosis can be confirmed by serological testing like Western blot assay or a RIBA strip immunoblot assay. Biopsy materials of postmortem tissues can be examined by RT-PCR test.

Prevention

No vaccine is yet available for human use. Trials for a human vaccine are underway in Asia but to date no SNV vaccine has been developed.

BIBLIOGRAPHY

1. Bryan RT, Doyle TJ, Molenae RL, et al. Hantavirus Pulmonary syndrome. Seminar in Paediatric infectious disease 1997;8:44-9.
2. MMWR Center for Disease Control and prevention. Update: Hantavirus pulmonary syndrome - United States 1993;42:816-20.
3. MMWR Center for disease control and prevention. Hantavirus pulmonary syndrome - Vermont 2000;50:603-5.

19 Chapter

Japanese Encephalitis and Other Viral Encephalitis

JK Dutta

A large number of viral agents have the capability to cause encephalitis. Primary neurotropic viruses include arbo virus, herpes virus and rabies virus. Few other incidental viral pathogens include retrovirus, orthomyxovirus, paramyxovirus, and adenovirus which may invade the CNS in a small proportion of patients **(Table 19.1)**.

Table 19.1: Arthropod-borne viruses which infect CNS

Family	*Members*
A. Bunyaviridae	1. California encephalitis
	2. La Crosse
	3. Crimean hemorrhagic fever
	4. Tensaw
	5. Rift Valley fever
B. Flaviviridae	1. Dengue
	2. Japanese B encephalitis
	3. Murray valley encephalitis
	4. Russian spring-summer encephalitis
	5. St. Louis encephalitis
	6. West nile encephalitis
	7. Yellow fever
	8. Ilheus
	9. Powassan
	10. Kumlinge
	11. Rocio
	12. Negishi
C. Togaviridae	1. Chikungunya
	2. Eastern equine encephalitis
	3. Venezuelan equine encephalitis
	4. Western equine encephalitis
	5. Thogoto
	6. Semliki forest disease
	7. O'nyong-nyong
D. Reovirdae	1. Colorado tick fever

In India, Japanese encephalitis is the most common form of viral encephalitis which causes epidemics over large parts of the country.

Global Incidence of Viral Encephalitis

In USA about 1000 to 2000 cases are reported every year. In a study in Beijing, etiological agents could be identified in 35 out of 97 cases. Enteroviruses were responsible for 15.4% cases. In 1996 to 1998, a study in Bangkok showed that in a group of 40 children 26 (65%) developed encephalitis due to viral agents; Dengue (8), Japanese encephalitis (JE) (6), Herpes simplex virus (HSV) (4), Human herpes virus 6 (HHV-6) (3), Mumps (2), Enterovirus (1), Varicella zoster virus (VZV) (1), and Rabies (1).

Arboviruses (arthropod-borne viruses) cause diseases primarily among vertebrates and arthropod vectors. Clinically important arboviruses belong to the Togaviridae and Bunyaviridae groups. Most of the arboviruses are spherical but few are rod shaped.

Several of these viruses cause acute encephalitis in man. Flaviviruses which often cause encephalitis are transmitted both by mosquitoes and tick; Japanese encephalitis (JE) virus is a mosquito-borne flavivirus. Other mosquito-borne flaviruses cause dengue-type 1,2,3,4, Murray valley encephalitis, West Nile encephalitis and others. Tick-borne flaviviruses cause Kyasanur Forest disease (KFD), Tick-borne encephalitis, Russian spring- Summer encephalitis and few other clinical illnesses.

Japanese encephalitis is prevalent in eastern Asia, Philippines, India, Japan and Indonesia. It was first reported in Japan in 1871. The Nakayam strain used in development of mouse brain inactivated virus vaccine was first isolated in 1935.

Etiology and Epidemiology

Japanese encephalitis is caused by flavivirus of group B arboviruses. It grows well in hamster and pig kidney cells. Pigs and ardeid birds (pond heron and cattle egrets) are the natural reservoirs. "Culex Tritaeniorhynchus" which breeds abundantly in rich fields is the main vector in north Asia and Japan. "Culex pipiens" is the usual vector in USSR whereas C Gelidus is responsible for transmission in Malayasia and C Vishnui group in India.

Scenario in India (Table 19.2)

In India JE was first recorded in Vellore and Pondicherry in south India in mid 1950s. In 1973 there was a major outbreak in Bankura and Bardhamandistricts of West Bengal. Outbreaks were also reported from Andhra Pradesh, Assam, Karnataka, Tamil Nadu, Uttar Pradesh and West Bengal in 1976. During 1988, a total of 4485 cases with 1413 deaths were recorded in Uttar Pradesh. A total of 1037 cases with 292 deaths were reported during 2002 from different states **(Table 19.3)**. Andhra Pradesh, Assam, Bihar, Goa, Karnataka, Manipur, Tamil Nadu, Uttar Pradesh and West Bengal are the highly affected areas.

Clinical Features

Japanese encephalitis is the most virulent of all encephalitis. It predominantly affects persons below 15 years of age. Most of the patients remain asymptomatic. Incubation period is 4 to 14 days. There is sudden onset in symptomatic cases with high fever, headache, stiff neck, coarse tremor, convulsion progressing to coma. Signs of acute meningoencephalitis develop quickly. Case fatality ranges from 20 to 50%. Outbreaks usually occur during monsoon and post-monsoon period when vector growth is high in rich fields. Permanent sequelae like mental impairment, motor neurone lesions and aphasia are commonly observed.

Laboratory Diagnosis

Diagnosis can be confirmed by detection of antigen of virus or by antibody testing.

Table 19.2: Scenario of Japanese encephalitis in India

Year	*Area*	*Comments*
1950s	Vellore and Pondicherry	First recorded
1973	Bankura and Bardhaman districts of West Bengal	First major outbreak
1976	Andhra Pradesh, Assam, Karnataka, Tamil Nadu, Uttar Pradesh, West Bengal	Wide outbreak
1988	Uttar Pradesh	Worst outbreak: 4485 cases, 1413 deaths.CFR-31.5%

Table 19.3: Japanese encephalitis in India during 2002

States	*Cases*	*Deaths*
Andhra Pradesh	18	3
Assam	472	150
Chandigarh	4	–
Delhi	1	–
Goa	11	–
Haryana	59	40
Karnataka	152	15
Maharashtra	27	12
Manipur	2	1
Punjab	10	2
Uttar Pradesh	281	69
Total	**1037**	**292**

The virus may be isolated and identified in CSF and in peripheral blood as well as in brain tissue after autopsy. Viral antigen may also be detected in brain tissues of autopsied patients by fluorescent antibody test. Antibodies to JE virus can be detected by hemagglutination inhibition (HI) test or IgM capture ELISA test. High level of IgM antibody in serum and rising titer of IgM antibody in paired sera are diagnostic of JE virus infection. Magnetic resonance imaging (MRI) has an important role in diagnosis and differential diagnosis of different neurological disorders.

Prevention and Control

Inactivated mouse brain vaccine is available in Japan, Korea, Thailand and India as well as in other parts of the world. Live attenuated primary hamster kidney cell and inactivated primary hamster kidney cell vaccines are manufactured and are available in China.

Mouse brain vaccine produced from Nakayama strain 1 ml is injected subcutaneously and 2nd dose of 1 ml is injected after one to four weeks. Booster dose should be administered after one year and additional booster doses every one to three years.

Control of vector is extremely important to prevent transmission to humans. Residual spraying of insecticides should be carried out before the onset of monsoon season so that vector growth can be adequately controlled. Since, pig is the natural reservoir of the virus there should not be piggeries close to the human habitation.

Other Neuro-viruses of Clinical Importance

Besides Japanese B encephalitis virus, several other viruses also cause important clinical illness. They are briefly mentioned below as it is beyond the scope of this monograph to give detail account of them.

Arenaviridae

Two major groups in this family are lymphocytic-choriomeningitis (LCM) and the Tacaribe complex. The LCM complex consists of lymphocytic choriomeningitis and Lassa viruses. The latter causes Lassa fever.

Bunyaviridae

California encephalitis and La Crosse (LAC) viruses are members of this family.

Phleboviruses

Rift valley fever (RVF) virus is the most important virus in this genus. An outbreak of this illness with encephalitis was reported in Egypt in 1979.

Coronaviridae

Several human serotypes of this family have been implicated in chronic bronchitis in adult humans.

Flaviviridae

It is now classified as an independent family. The mosquito-borne viruses of this family include Japanese B encephalitis (JE), West Nile (WN), St Louis encephalitis (SLE), Murray valley encephalitis (MVE) and Rocio viruses.

The tick-borne viruses of the family are Russian spring-summer encephalitis (RSSE), Louping ill, Negishi and Powassan encephalitis virus.

Herpetoviridae

The following members of this group cause CNS infection in humans particularly, among those with acquired immuno deficiency syndrome (AIDS). They include herpes simplex virus 1 and 2, human cytomegalovirus (HCMV), varicella-zoster virus (VZV), Epstein-Barr virus (EBV), human herpesvirus 6, 7 and 8.

Paramyxoviridae

Important members of this family which cause human illness are measles, mumps, parainfleunza (Types 1–4) and Respiratory Syncytial virus.

Enteroviruses

The viruses of this genus which are important CNS pathogens in humans include polio virus and Coxsackie virus.

Rhabdoviridae

This family is divided into genera Lyssa virus and Vesiculo virus. Rabies virus is a member of the genus lyssa virus.

Alphavirus

It is a member of the family Togaviridae. These viruses include Eastern Equine Encephalitis (EEE) virus, Venezuela equine encephalitis (VEE), Western equine encephalitis (WEE) viruses and others. Chikungunya virus is also known to cause neurological complications.

Rubivirus

The sole member of rubivirus genus is rubella virus which causes rubella in humans.

Kyasanur Forest Disease Virus

It is a flavivirus antigenically related to West Nile, Tick-borne encephalitis (TBE) and Omsk hemorrhagic fever (OHF) viruses. Kyasanur forest disease was first described in 1957 in Kyasanur Forest of Mysore in India.

BIBLIOGRAPHY

1. C D Alert. National Institute of Communicable Diseases, Delhi 2003;7:1-8.
2. Hardas UD, Pathak AA, Jahagirdar UL. Virological studies in encephalitis. Ind J Pediatr 1976;43:270-71.
3. Kumar R, Mathur A, Singh KB, et al. Clinical sequelae of Japanese encephalitis in Children. Ind J Med Res 1993;97:9-13.
4. Kumar R. Viral encephalitis. Paediatrics today 2000;3:34-41.
5. Kumar R,Agarwal SP, Wakhlu I, et al. Japanese encephalitis-an encephalomyelitis. Ind Pediatr 1991;28:1525-28.
6. Male D, Rezaie P. Colonisation of the human central nervous system by microglia; the role of chemokines and vascular adhesion molecules. Prog Brain Res 2001;132:81-93.
7. Tiroumourougane SV, Raghava P, Srinivasan S. Japanese viral encephalitis. Post Grad Med J 2002;78:205-15.

20 Chapter Hepatitis C

JK Dutta, Madhumala Giri

Hepatitis A and B viruses were identified in 1960s and 1970s. Thereafter another agent named initially as Non-A, Non-B virus was reported to be responsible for same disease in blood transfusion recipients and drug users. This was later named as Hepatitis C virus (HCV) which is a single stranded RNA virus of the Flaviviridae family. HCV is genetically diverse. There are at least six major genotypes each with more than 50 subtypes. Coinfection with more than one genotype may occur.

Prevalence

Serology of HCV is positive in 1.8% of population in USA. Male persons in the age group 30 to 49 years are the common victims. Worldwide, more than one million cases are reported each year. Hepatitis C virus is now the major cause of cirrhosis, end-stage liver disease and cancer of liver.

Transmission

Major routes of transmission include transfusion of blood and blood products from infected donors, use of drug by contaminated apparatus or through transplantation. As many as one-third of HIV infected persons are known to be coinfected with HCV. Transmission from patients to health care workers and vice versa has been reported. Tattooing, acupuncture and human bites have been associated with HCV infection. Intranasal cocaine use is associated with positive HCV serology. Sexual transmission is frequent both among commercial sex workers and casual sex partners. Prenatal transmission from HCV infected mother to infant is also known.

Clinical Features

The incubation period varies from two weeks to six months with an average of seven weeks. Some individuals may remain asymptomatic even for decades. In few infected persons the illness starts with nausea, vomiting, right sided abdominal pain, and weight loss. Jaundice appears in about 30% of symptomatic adults.

About 85 to 90% of persons who have acute attacks pass on to a chronic stage. In about 20 to 30% persons with chronic HCV infection cirrhosis develops with portal hypertension, ascites, esophageal varices with bleeding. Cryoglobulinemia develops in some patients. Hepatocellular carcinoma may develop in some patients with HCV related cirrhosis.

Diagnosis

Enzyme immune assay (EIA) is used for screening for anti-HCV antibody. Recombinant immunoblot assay (RIBA) is a suitable test for confirmation of diagnosis. Polymerase chain reaction (PCR) can directly detect HCV RNA.

Treatment and Prevention

Alpha interferon treatment is indicated for patients with chronic hepatitis C infection. Treatment should be started in a dose of 3×106 units three times a week subcutaneously for six months. Addition of ribavirin in a dosage of 800 to 1200 mg daily has been found to improve the efficacy of interferon. Hemolysis may develop in some patients as a side effect of ribavirin therapy.

No vaccine is yet available for prevention. Counseling is essential for drug users who should stop use of drugs. Razor, tooth brush or syringe/needles should not be shared. Sex should be practiced with faithful partners only.

BIBLIOGRAPHY

1. Alter HJ, Purcell RH, Shih JW, et al. Detection of antibody to hepatitis C in prospectively followed transfusion recipients with acute and chronic non-A, non-B hepatitis. N Engl J Med 1989;321:1944-1500.
2. Bronowicki JP, Verhard V, Botte C, et al. Patient to patient transmission of hepatitis C virus during colonoscopy. N Engl J Med 1997;337:237-40.
3. Esteban JI, Games J, Martell M, Cabot B, et al. Transmission of hepatitis C virus by a cardiac surgeon. N Engl J Med 1996;334:550-60.
4. Lawrence SP. Advances in the treatment of hepatitis C. Advance in Int Med 2000;45:65-105.

21 Chapter

Ebola Hemorrhagic Fever, Rift Valley Fever and Nipah Virus Infection

JK Dutta

Ebola Hemorrhagic Fever

In January 1995, a man died of bloody diarrhea in Zaire (Democratic Republic of Congo). He was diagnosed as a case of shigella infection. By April 1995 some nursing staff at the Maternity Hospital in Kuwait also suffered from similar illness. A number of physicians and nurses subsequently acquired the same infection in the hospital. So for investigation, samples were sent to CDC, USA where Ebola Virus was isolated.

Virus

Ebola virus is a member of the family Filoviridae. Ebola virus has four subtypes; it is rod-shaped with brush-like spikes protruding from the anterior membrane. Person-to-person transmission is known to occur. Ebola virus was named after a river in North-West Zaire.

By January 23, 2001, Ebola cases were reported from Democratic Republic of Congo bordering Uganda. In November 2001, an outbreak was recorded in Gabon. Asymptomatic human infection has been observed recently. Natural reservoir of Ebola virus has not yet been identified.

Clinical Manifestation

The disease is spread by close contact with sick persons suffering from the disease. Incubation period is 4 to 10 days. There is sudden onset with fever, myalgia, severe frontal headache with bradycardia and conjunctivitis. A maculopapular rash may appear around 5th day of illness. Petechiae, ecchymoses or frank bleeding may occur. Most patients die in a stage of shock and coma. Case fatality rate is high (65–90%). No specific treatment is available. Barrier-nursing and supportive measures should be provided for management of the cases.

RIFT VALLEY FEVER

It is a zoonotic disease caused by Rift Valley fever virus in Africa. From the animals like sheep and cattle, it is transmitted to man by mosquitoes. It causes hemorrhagic fever which may be followed by death. In the year 2000, the disease spread from Africa to Yemen and the Kingdom of Saudi Arabia (KSA). Rift valley fever virus causes at least four different clinical syndromes: Febrile-myalgic syndrome, hemorrhagic fever, retinal vasculitis and encephalitis.

Treatment

Ribavirin intravenously can be used for treatment of hemorrhagic fever caused by Rift Valley fever virus.

Prevention

A formalin-inactivated vaccine is available which can be used for prevention among laboratory workers and veterinarians.

NIPAH VIRUS INFECTION

In Malaysia and Singapore cases of febrile encephalitis and respiratory distress were investigated in 1999 among persons exposed to pigs. On laboratory testing a paramyxovirus was identified. This virus is now named as Nipah virus (previously named as Hendra like virus). Source of infection to human is exposure to pigs. Man-to-man transmission has not yet been documented.

BIBLIOGRAPHY

1. Center for disease control and prevention. Update: outbreak of Rift Valley fever - Saudi Arabia. MMWR 2000;49:982-5.
2. Clua KB, Bellini WJ, Rota PA, Harcount BH, et al. Nipah virus: a recently emergent deadly paramyxovirus. Science 2000;288:1432-35.
3. House JA, Turell MJ, Melus CA. Rift Valley fever: Present status and risk to the Western Hemisphere. Ann N Y Acad Sc 1992;653:233-42.
4. Shope RE, Peters CJ, Davies FG. The spread of Rift valley fever and approaches to its control. Bulletin of World Health Organization 1982;60:299-304.
5. World Health Organization (2001). Outbreak news. Ebola, Uganda (upadate). Weekly Epidemiology Record 76,1.
6. World Health Organization (December 2000). Ebola haemorrhagic fever. Fact sheet (no. 103).

22 Chapter Rabies in Canada and USA

JK Dutta

RABIES IN CANADA

Canada has remained free from rabies since 1985. However a patient died of rabies on 6th October 2000 in Quebec.

A 9-year-old boy developed fever and pain in left upper arm on 22nd September, 2000. Later, on 28th September he had hydrophobia, aerophobia, tremor, myoclonus, visual hallucination and hypersalivation. The patient was treated in a children's hospital. Several laboratory investigations were carried out because of presumptive diagnosis of rabies.

History

On 28th August 2000, the brother of the patient found a bat in the bathroom which had difficulty in flying. The bat was removed by his father. The same night he and his brother slept in rural cottage when his parents found a bat in the kitchen. Approximately three days later the patient contacted his mother and showed her an erythematous area with a small central laceration of almost 2 cm size on the left upper arm. No treatment was given to him then. He developed rabies and died on 6th October.

Laboratory Investigation

Nuchal skin biopsy material was examined by Direct Fluorescent Antibody Test which yielded positive result for rabies. Saliva, tears, and skin biopsy examined gave positive result for rabies by Reverse Transcriptase Polymerase Chain Reaction. Molecular analysis of the virus revealed a rabies variant associated with silver-haired (*Lasionycteris noctivagans*) and eastern pipistrelle (*Pipistrellus subflavus*) bats. Hence diagnosis of rabies was confirmed as the cause of his death.

RABIES IN USA: PAST AND CURRENT STATUS

Human rabies is extremely rare in USA. However, every year 16,000 to 39,000 persons are assessed. Between 1980 and 1997, approximately 25 to 247 cases of rabies were reported every year among dogs. Rabies among wildlife especially raccoons, skunks and bats has become more prevalent since 1950s which accounts for more than 85% of all reported cases.

During the year 1998 only one person died of laboratory confirmed rabies in USA. Rabies was reported among 7961 animals during the year out of which the disease was identified in 113 dogs, 282 cats and the rest were in other species of animals. 32 deaths from human rabies have been recorded since 1990. Out of them bite by bat was established in two cases only.

Current Status (2000s)

During the period 2000 and onwards some case of rabies were reported in USA. On 15 September 2000, a 49-year-old man in California developed pain in right arm. Later he developed dysphagia, hypersalivation and became agitated. He developed respiratory failure and died on 20th September. The patient did not report contact with any bat. Diagnosis of rabies was confirmed by direct fluorescent antibody test of material from skin and cornea and also by reverse transcriptase polymerase chain reaction of saliva.

A 54-year-old man who had resided in Ghana arrived and stayed in New York. On 22nd September 2000 he developed pain in abdomen and was treated for suspected bowel obstruction. There was swelling in right lumbar area along with vomiting, delirium, agitation and he died of respiratory failure. Diagnosis of rabies was established by laboratory tests. Direct fluorescent antibody test of skin biopsy material gave positive result for rabies. Reverse transcriptase polymerase chain reaction of saliva was also positive for rabies.

A 26-year-old man in Georgia developed intractable vomiting and hematemesis on 3rd October 2000. He had anisocoria and hypersalivation. On 9th October he developed cardiac arrhythmia and respiratory as well as renal failure. He died on 10th October. He had informed coworkers that bats from the attic had entered his living quarters and landed on him while he was asleep. Diagnosis of rabies was confirmed by direct fluoresent antibody test on postmortem examination.

In Minnesota a 47-year-old man visited a local clinic on 14th October 2000 because of pain in the right arm. Later he developed anisocorea, flaccid paralysis with sensory loss in right upper arm and hyporeflexia in the left upper extremity. He also developed acute respiratory failure and died on 25th October. Three days later, one of his friends told that he had been awakened by a bat. He killed the bat but was himself bitten by the bat.

Diagnosis of rabies was confirmed by positive direct fluorescent antibody test and reverse transcriptase-polymerase chain reaction of skin biopsy material and saliva.

In Wisconsin a 69-year-old man developed chest discomfort, numbness and tingling. Two days later he had dysphagia, diaphoresis and delirium.

He was treated for suspected herpes encephalitis. He developed renal insufficiency and died.

Diagnosis of rabies was confirmed by rapid fluorescent focus inhibition test (RFFIT) for rabies antibodies. Negri bodies were detected in brain tissues after postmortem examination. It came to light later that he had removed bats from his house with bare hands.

Rabies in 2004

In June-July 2004, center for disease control and prevention, confirmed diagnosis of rabies in three recipients of transplanted organs and their common donor in USA. The donor was a man from Arkansas. After death his lungs, liver, kidneys were recovered. The liver recipient had end-stage liver disease. Twenty-one days after transplantation, the recipient developed diffuse encephalitis and died.

A female patient in end-stage renal disease developed cerebral edema and died few days after receiving a kidney transplant.

Another male kidney transplant recipient developed neurological manifestations 27 days after transplantation and died. Diagnosis of rabies in the donor and all the recipients was confirmed by laboratory investigations at Baylor University Medical Center (BUMC) in Dallas, Texas.

A Case of Recovery in Wisconsin

A girl aged 15 years was bitten by a bat on her left index finger during church service in Wisconsin, USA in October 2004. The wound was cleaned but no rabies vaccine was administered. She had not received any pre-exposure vaccination also.

About a month after the bat bite she became ill. Rabies virus specific antibodies were detected in the serum and CSF of the girl. The attending physician obtained the consent of the parents and kept her in drug-induced coma for seven days and used some antiviral drugs. She improved steadily towards recovery.

BIBLIOGRAPHY

1. MMWR. December 15, 2000/49(49):1115. Public Health Dispatch: Human Rabies- Quebec, Canada 2000.
2. MMWR. July 9, 2004/53 (dispatch): 1 update: Investigation of rabies infections in organ donor and Transplant Recipients- Alabama, Arkansas, Oklahoma and Texas 2004.

23 Chapter

Dengue Fever

JK Dutta

Dengue fever (DF) is widely distributed in the world in tropical and subtropical regions. It is prevalent in South-East-Asia, the Pacific, East and West Africa, the Caribbean and the Americas. Transovarian spread has been documented. Immunity is antibody mediated.

Epidemics of the disease became widespread and more frequent in the 18th and 19th centuries. The epidemic has risen dramatically since 1980s. These outbreaks and extensions to the Americas and South-East-Asia resulted from an increase in human and commercial traffic.

Etiology

The causative agent is an RNA virus belonging to the family flaviviridae and is an arthropod-borne (Arbo virus) virus. Man is the main reservoir of infection. However it has been shown that monkey is the jungle reservoir in Malaysia and Africa.

Four dengue serotypes are known and designated as DEN-1, DEN-2, DEN-3, DEN-4. Besides *Aedes aegypti*, several other mosquito species are known to transmit the virus. They are *Aedes albopictus, polynesiensis* and some forms of *Aedes scutellaris*.

Epidemiology

Globally there are about 50 to 100 million cases of DF and 4,50,000 cases of dengue hemorrhagic fever (DHF) every year. In 1995, about 7000 cases of DHF were reported in Americas. The first epidemic was reported in Philippines during 1953 to 55. By mid 1970s DHF reached epidemic proportion in South-East-Asia including several countries like India, Pakistan, Sri Lanka, Maldives, etc. 886 patients of Dengue were admitted at All India Institute of Medical Sciences, New Delhi alone in an outbreak in 2006.

First Cases of Dengue in Americas

In the summer of 1995, twelve male persons of Texas participated in a construction assistance mission in Reynosa, a Mexican town across the border in Tamaulipas state. Out of them three became ill with fever, headache, vomiting and one had enlarged liver and gradually declining thrombocytopenia. On serological examination DEN-4 viral isolates were detected in all three patients. During next two months during surveillance in South Texas areas, 29 were identified with dengue. There was abundance of *Aedes aegypti* mosquitoes in the area which was the vector of dengue. Cases numbering 2706 were reported from the city of Tamaulipas in Reynosa state.

Clinical Features

A general classification of disease includes mild dengue fever, dengue hemorrhagic fever (DHF) and dengue shock syndrome (DSS). In some patients the infection may remain asymptomatic while in others the infection may result in critical illness.

There is fever, severe headache, joint pain, weakness and skin rash. Incubation period is 5 to 8 days. Classic dengue is followed by general weakness which lasts several weeks. Cough, headache and vomiting accompany fever. A relative bradycardia is common during febrile stage.

Several types of rash have been observed. Initially diffuse flushing, mottling or pin point eruptions may be observed on face and chest. Around third or fourth day of onset there may be maculopapular or scarlitiform rash. Rash subsides towards the end of febrile period.

All four dengue serotypes are capable of causing dengue or dengue hemorrhagic fever (DHF) depending on the immune status. DHF occurs usually under the age of 16 years of age. Dengue shock syndrome (DSS) can proceed quickly to death unless properly treated.

Diagnosis

Diagnosis can be confirmed by serological tests for antibodies, virus isolation or by detection of dengue antigen by polymerase chain reaction (PCR). Anti-dengue lgM and lgG antibodies can be detected by Enzyme-linked Immunosorbant Assay (ELISA). Antibody capture (MAC ELISA) is a relatively new but useful diagnostic test. Hemagglutination inhibition test with fourfold rise in antibody in paired sera is also helpful for confirmation of diagnosis but it needs long time (2–3 weeks).

Treatment

Replacement of fluid and electrolytes by plasma, plasma expanders or electrolyte solution is an urgent need. Aspirin is contraindicated which may precipitate Reye's syndrome or bleeding. Acetaminophen may be used with caution. Thrombocytopenia does not require platelet transfusion unless associated with spontaneous bleeding.

Prevention

No vaccine is yet available for prevention of dengue. Mosquito control is the urgent need as a preventive measure. In tropical countries travelers should use aerosol "Bomb" type insecticides to kill indoor mosquitoes and use diethyltoluamide (DEET) as mosquito repellant on exposed skin and on protective clothing. Long sleeved clothes should be used to avoid mosquito bite.

BIBLIOGRAPHY

1. Center for Disease Control and Prevention. Dengue fever at the US-Mexico Border. MMWR 1996;45:841-2.
2. Center for Disease Control and Prevention. Underdiagnosed dengue-Laredo, Texas 1999. MMWR 2001;50:57-9.
3. Chye JK, Lim CT, Ng KB. Vertical transmission of Dengue. Clin Infect Dis 1997;25:1374-7.
4. Jacobs M. Dengue: Emergence as a global public health problem and prospects for control. Trans Roy Soc Trop Med Hyg 2000;94:7-8.
5. Mc Bride WJH, Bielefeldt-Ohmann H. Dengue viral infections: Pathogenesis and epidemiology. Microb and infection 2000;2:1041-60.
6. Moore CG, Mitchell CJ. Aedes albopictious in the United States. Ten year presence and public health implications. Emerg Inf Dis 1997;3:329-34.
7. World Health Organization. Dengue/dengue haemorrhagic fever: Situation in 2000. Weekly Epidemiological Record 2000;75:193-6.
8. World Health Organization-Dengue haemorrhagic fever. Diagnosis treatment, prevention and control, 2nd edn. 1997 Geneva.

24 Chapter

Malaria: A Re-emerging Infection in USA

JK Dutta

Malaria is a worldwide health problem with about 300 to 500 million cases reported every year out of which about 2.7 million die. It is endemic in nearly 100 countries. It has re-emerged in USA now, though the disease had been eradicated by the middle of 20th century. Although usual mode of infection is bite by infected female *Anopheles* mosquitoes, in rare instance the disease may develop after transfusion of blood and sometimes by congenital transmission. Due to increasing international air travel and drug resistance, imported cases among travelers and immigrants are now more common.

RE-EMERGENCE OF MALARIA IN USA

On August 19 1999, an 11-year-old boy living in Suffolk County, New York developed fever with rigor, abdominal pain and vomiting. Examination of thick and thin peripheral blood smears at the New York State Department of Health and Center for Disease Control and Prevention confirmed presence of *plasmodium vivax*. The patient was adequately treated with antimalarial drugs. This was indeed a case of locally acquired malaria in USA.

Re-emergence of malaria is a public health hazard in USA now. Every year about 1000 cases of malaria are reported in US, most of which are among travelers, immigrants and refugees. Several factors contribute to the re-emergence of the disease like easy international air travel, population growth, immigration, global warming, resistance of the parasite to drugs, resistance of the vectors to insecticides and disruption due to natural disasters. Mosquito vectors feeding on infected individuals spread the disease.

In the last decade malaria has been reported from many areas in USA which include Georgia, Vermont, Pennsylvania, New York, Minnesota, Texas, Florida and few others. In USA, most of the locally acquired cases are caused by *plasmodium vivax* which produces a mild clinical illness. Among the imported cases, the infection is caused by *P. vivax* and

P. falciparum. Most of the infection imported to USA is from Africa, India, Central America and the Caribbean. The largest number of cases is reported from California, New York, Florida and Illinois.

The situation regarding malaria is getting worse in many parts of the world. Treatment is becoming difficult and ineffective due to increasing resistance of the parasite to antimalarial drugs.

Diagnosis of Malaria

Both thick and thin smears of peripheral blood should be examined (Giemsa stain). Species detection of the parasite is easy in thin smears. New technology of diagnosis is based on an antigen-capture dip-stick methodology using a monoclonal antibody to *P. falciparum* histidine-rich protein-2. Dipstick method is a potentially quick and accurate method of diagnosis. Polymerase chain reaction (PCR) test detects the malaria parasites directly. Fluorescent dye is used in Kawarnoto technique to detect the parasite.

Treatment and Chemoprophylaxis

In USA several drugs are available for treatment of malaria. Chloroquine though a standard drug for treatment of malaria often fails to be effective because of drug resistance by the parasite. Resistant case may be treated with quinine, doxycycline, mefloquine, primaquin or malrone. Artemisin and proguanil may also be used. Where there is multi-drug resistance oral quinine may be combined with an antibiotic. For treatment of severe cases of malaria, quinine can be administered intravenously.

In quinine-resistant severe *falciparum* malaria, WHO recommends artemesinin combination therapy (ACT) in following dosage:

Artesunate 2.4 mg/kg stat IV, followed by same dose at 12 and 24 hours, then daily for 7 days + Doxycycline 3 mg/kg daily for 7 days.

A new agent triclosan has been developed for treatment of malaria. It acts by inhibiting enoyl-ACP reductase of *P. falciparum*.

Chemoprophylaxis is essential for local residents as well as for travelers. It should begin one week before travel and be discontinued four weeks after the last possible exposure. Efforts are in progress to develop an effective vaccine for prevention of the disease.

Chloroquine can be used provided there is no known resistance to this drug. Mefloquine resistance is known. So doxycycline should be used as alternative to mefloquine. Sulfadoxine-pyrimethamine can be used for self medication in areas when medical care is not quickly available.

For prevention mosquito net should be used. Mosquito breeding should be prevented by eliminating collection of water, using insecticides and increasing public awareness by health education. Impregnated bed nets are particularly useful since they are impregnated with insecticides.

BIBLIOGRAPHY

1. Center for Disease Control and Prevention. Probable locally acquired mosquito-transmitted *plasmodium vivax* infection- Suffolk County, New York. MMWR 1999;49:495-8.
2. Center for Disease Control and Prevention. Microscopic procedures for diagnosing malaria MMWR. 2001;50(SS-05):19-20.
3. Center of Disease Control and Prevention. Malaria deaths following inappropriate malaria chemoprophylaxis-United States 2001. MMWR 2001; 50:597-9.
4. Surolia N, Surolia A. Triclosan offers protection against blood stages of malaria by inhibiting enoyl-ACP reductase of *plasmodium falciparum*. Nat Med 2001;7:167-73.
5. Warhurst DC. A molecular marker for chloroquine resistant *falciparum* malaria. N Engl J Med 2001;344:299-302.
6. Zucker J. Changing pattern of autochthonous malaria transmission in the United States: A review of recent outbreaks. Em Inf Dis 1996;2:37-63.

25 Chapter

Emerging Therapy for a Re-emerging Disease: Combination Therapy for Malaria—A Brief Outline

TK Dutta

Malaria has remained a problematic infection in India for several centuries. The disease has been discussed in detail in ancient literature like "Charaka Samhita". The Government of India started the National Malaria Eradication Program (NMEP) in 1958. In 1976, NMEP recorded highest number of cases numbering 6.45 million though the number had dropped to 50,000 cases per year since 1961.

Even today malaria is a major public health problem. An estimated 300 to 500 million cases are reported every year. Multi-drug resistance of malaria parasites is a serious hazard today. So combination therapy has emerged as a suitable alternative for treatment of malaria.

ANTIMALARIA DRUGS

There are several families of drugs which can be used for treatment of malaria. Chloroquine is a cheap and effective drug. Based on the gain obtained by combined drug therapy in tuberculosis and leprosy the combination therapy is now being used for treatment of malaria.

Antimalaria combination therapy is defined as the simultaneous use of two or more blood schizonticidal drugs with independent mode of action and thus unrelated by biochemical targets in the parasite.

Two broad groups of combinations include:

1. Artemisin based combination therapy (ACT)
2. Nonartemisin based combination therapy (Non-ACT)

Since 2001, the World Health Organization has recommended use of artemisin based combintion therapy (ACT) in areas experiencing resistance to older drugs.

However, cost remains a major barrier to ACT therapy since ACTs may cost up to 20 times as much as older medications. Malaria parasite can develop resistance to artemisin; resistance can be produced by mutation of SERCA. SERCA is a calcium pump in the endoplasmic reticulum. Nonetheless, it is also suggested that mitochondria is the major target for artemisin and its analogs.

Uncomplicated *P. Falciparum* Malaria

Artemisin Based Combination Therapy (ACT)

Currently there are four artemisin based combination therapy (ACTs) which have been recommended by WHO for treatment of uncomplicated *P. falciparum* malaria. They are:

a. Artemisin + Lumefantrine (AL)
b. Artemisin + Mefloquine (AS + MQ)
c. Artemisin + Sulfadoxine-Pyrimethamine (AS + SP)
d. Artesunate + Amodiaquine (AS + AQ)

All the four regimens are effective and superior to monotherapy for malaria. Second-line treatment: Artesunate + Doxycycline

Non-artemisin Based Combination Therapy (Non-ACT)

a. Sulfadoxine - Pyrimethamine + Chloroquine (SP + CQ)
b. Sulfadoxine - Pyrimethamine + Amodiaquine (SP + AQ)
c. Qunine + Tetracycline/Doxycycline
d. Quinine + Clindamycin

Complicated or Severe *Falciparum* Malaria

Artesunate (intravenous) + Doxycycline

Few other combinations like dihydroartemisinin-piperaquine are also highly efficacious and less expensive. Atovaquone with proguanil and fosmidomycin with clindamycin also show promising results. They however await WHO recommendation.

In February 2002 a new drug called "G25" has been found to cure malaria in test primates. In 2005 an oral therapy called "TE3" or "Te3" has been found to be an effective antimalarial agent.

Multi-drug resistant malaria parasites have urged the therapists to introduce combination regimens. Role of monotherapy for malaria is now limited.

BIBLIOGRAPHY

1. Kremsner PG, Krishna S. Antimalaria combinations. Lancet 2004;364:285-94.
2. Mohapatra MK, Panda BK, Das ST. Cerebellar ataxia in falciparum malaria - a report of two cases. Ind J Malariol 2000;37(1-2):46-8.
3. Panda M, Mohapatra A. Malaria control-An overview in India. J Hum Ecol 2004;15:101-4.
4. Philips RS. Current status of malaria and potential for control. Clinical Microbiology Reviews 2001;14:208-26.
5. Sharma VP. Re-emergence of malaria in India. Ind J Med Res 1996;103:26-45.
6. South-East Asian Quinine Artesunates Malaria Trial (SEAQUAMT) group. Artesunate versus quinine for treatment of severe *falciparum* malaria: A randomized trial. Lancet 2005;366:717-25.

7. Surolia N, Surolia AC. Triclosan offers protection against blood stages of malaria by inhibiting enoyl - ACP reductase of *plasmodium falciparum*. Nature Medicine. 2001;7:167-73.
8. WHO 2000, WHO Expert committee on malaria. Twentieth report World Health Organization, Geneva. Technical Report Series No. 892.
9. WHO Geneva, Guidelines for treatment of malaria. World Health Organization; 2006.pp.1-253.

26 Chapter Hydatidosis/Cystic *Echinococcosis*

Amitabh Giri, Madhumala Giri, BK Giri

INTRODUCTION

Hydatidosis otherwise known as cystic *echinococcosis* is commonly known as dog tapeworm or small tapeworm. Humans are infected predominantly by two species. The cystic *echinococcosis* or cystic hydatid disease is caused by *Echinococcus granulosus*. The alveolar *echinococcus* or alveolar hydatid disease is caused by *Echinococcus multilocularis.*

Distribution

The infection with *E. granulosus* although occurs worldwide, the disease occurs more commonly in temperate climates than in tropical areas. It is more commonly found in countries where cattle and sheep raising is an important industry and thus there is close association between man, sheep and dog. Hence, it is more commonly seen in South and Central America, Asia, Europe, Africa, Middle East, Russia and China. It was thought earlier that hydatidosis was not so common in India. With the advent of newer diagnostic imaging tools and serological tests more occurrences are being noticed in India.

History, Mode of Infection and Pathogenesis

Man harbors the larval form. The adult worm is found in the small intestine of the dog and other canine animals. Hartman in the year 1965 discovered the adult worm, and the larval form was discovered by Goeze in 1782.

Life Cycle

The life cycle of the worm is completed in two hosts:

1. *Definitive host:* Dogs and other canine animals like fox and wolves act as definitive hosts. The adult worm lives in the small intestine of those canine animals. They discharge large number of eggs in their feces.
2. *Intermediate host:* Sheep, cattle, pig and man act as the intermediate host, where the larval stage occurs and it finally causes the hydatid cyst.

The canine animals (the dog being the optimum definitive host), which harbor the adult worms pass large numbers of eggs in their feces. These are swallowed by the sheep and cattle while grazing in the fields. The eggs are also ingested by man, especially by children through different modes:

1. Intimate contact with infected dogs like handling and fondling
2. By sharing food from the same utensils with the dog
3. By ingesting uncooked vegetables contaminated with infected feces.

The eggs after getting ingested by the intermediate hosts are hatched into hexacanth embryos in the duodenum. The embryos bore through the intestinal wall and enter into the portal system and then are carried to the liver. Most of them get arrested in the sinusoidal capillaries of the liver. The liver acts as the first filter for the embryos. Thus about 62% of the cases occur in the liver. Some of them pass through the hepatic capillaries to enter the pulmonary circulation where they get arrested. The lung acts as the second filter causing about 20% of the cases. However, a few of them also escape the second filter to enter the general circulation. The embryos while circulating in the general circulation get lodged in various organs of the body and can involve almost all organs of the body, e.g. kidney, heart, bone, muscle, spleen, pancreas, brain and urogenital organs.

Clinical Features

Hydatid disease usually takes several years to become symptomatic as the rate of growth in man is very slow. The average growth of the hydatid cyst is approximately 5 to 10 mm per year. The early phase of the infestation is usually asymptomatic. The symptomatology depends upon the size and site of the developing cyst. The growing cyst may cause pressure effect on the adjacent organs and vascular channel and thereby cause symptoms. It can also cause symptom due to extrinsic pressure causing vascular compromise to the organs. Symptoms can also be attributed to hypersensitivity reactions caused by the fluid within the cyst getting ruptured to the adjacent areas which may cause anaphylactic shock and death. Occasionally, the anaphylactic shock may be the first presenting symptom. The cyst can get infected and cause acute symptoms, which needs early surgical intervention. Some people who are infested may remain latent for several years and may get detected only at autopsy.

Liver being the first filter of its life cycle, the first symptom can be hepatomegaly with or without a palpable mass in the right upper quadrant and epigastric region. It can present as epigastric pain, nausea, vomiting and occasionally cholestatic jaundice. It can cause Budd-Chiari syndrome due to the pressure effect over the hepatic venous channel or inferior vena cava. When there are multiple cysts or the cyst is too large and is inoperable, it can lead to hepatic compromise and may lead to biliary cirrhosis. Sometimes the cyst can rupture into the adjacent gallbladder or the biliary channel and cause biliary colic, cholangitis, obstructive jaundice and pancreatitis **(Fig. 26.1)**.

The next common organ to be affected is the lung, which acts as the second filter **(Fig. 26.2)**. In infected person, it causes chronic cough, hemoptysis, bilioptysis, lung abscess, pleuritis and very rarely lung embolism.

Hydatid cyst can affect the cardiac muscles and pericardium and present as cardiac tumor and pericardial effusion. Rarely cardiac tamponade and complete heart block leading to death have been reported.

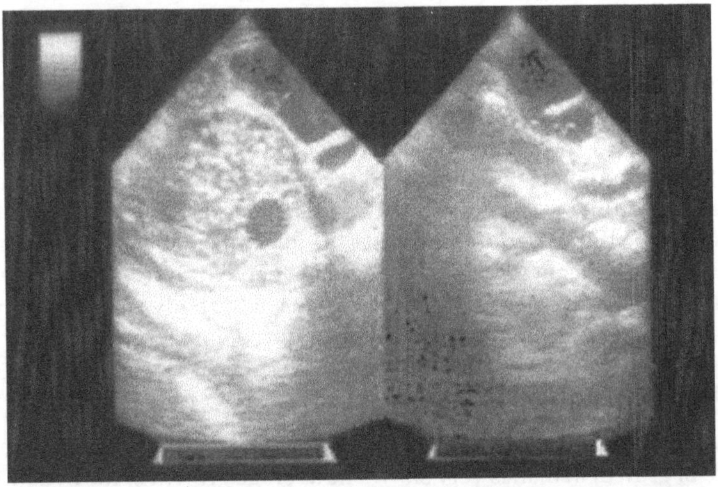

Fig. 26.1: Shows a hepatic hydatid cyst very close to the gallbladder which has ruptured into the gallbladder with daughter cysts in the gallbladder lumen

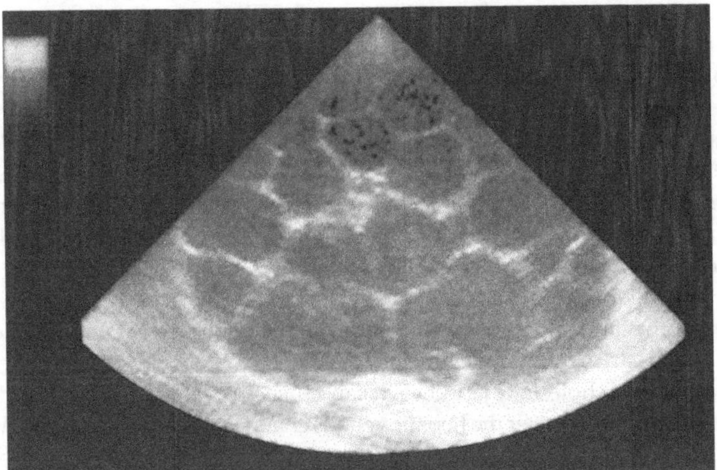

Fig. 26.2: Shows a hydatid cyst with sands in the left lung

It also affects the brain causing pressure symptoms and convulsive disorders. When the spine is involved by the cyst, it causes neurological symptoms depending on its location and level of compression. Rarely, it is a cause of stroke in young patients.

The spleen, kidneys, muscles and bones, uterus, ovaries are rarely involved and present as mass in the respective organs and symptoms appear due to pressure effect caused in the organs and the adjacent tissues.

Majority of the patients with cystic *echinococcosis* have single organ involvement. But in about 10 to 15% of patients it is simultaneously seen in two or more organs. Ultrasonogram may shows presence of hydatid cysts simultaneously in the liver and lung in the same person **(Fig. 26.2)**. Although, liver acts as the first filter, very rarely it has been seen to bypass liver and lung and affect other organs.

Diagnosis

Clinically, hydatidosis is suspected by the presence of a mass in the affected area or organ when further investigations are warranted.

Diagnostic imaging procedures along with serological tests clinch the diagnosis. Ultrasonography is the modality of choice for the diagnosis of *Echinococcosis*. However, false positivity rate is about 10% when it becomes difficult to differentiate between the hydatid cyst and simple benign hepatic cyst. The ultrasound diagnostic feature is the presence of a solitary large cyst with separation of germinal layer from the surrounding host capsule. Other diagnostic feastures are collapsed cyst (water lily sign **(Fig. 26.3)**, daughter cysts (cyst-in-cyst/cart-wheel appearance) (**Fig. 26.4**), calcification of the wall of the cyst or totally calcified cyst.

Hydatid 'sands' **(Fig. 26.2)** within the cyst are said as pathognomonic; however, in contrast it is also seen in simple hepatic cyst. High resolution sonography (HRSG) with higher frequency probes are of great help in diagnosing musculo-skeletal and ocular hydatid cysts. Ultrasonography is also of great help in the follow-up of treated cases.

- *Chest Skiagram:* Shows a homogenously opaque shadow having well defined and smooth margin in cases of lung hydatid cyst. CT scan of the lung shows the characteristic image of hydatid cyst as seen in the ultrasonography.
- *CT* and *MRI* scan are superior diagnostic tools when the brain, spinal cord or vertebrae are affected causing neurological symptoms.
- *ERCP* (Endoscopic retrograde cholangio-pancreaticography) has got added value when there is suspicion of rupture of the hepatic hydatid cyst into the biliary tract. However, a good sonography in an expert hand can avoid lengthy and expensive interventional procedures and its complications too.

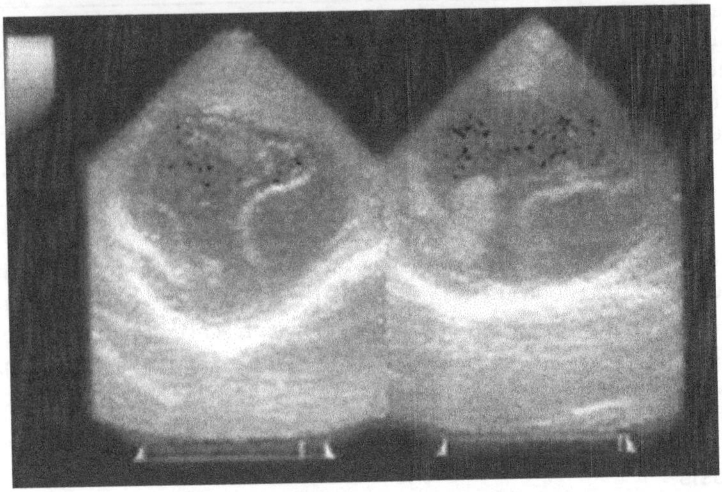

Fig. 26.3: Shows collapsed cyst (water lily sign)

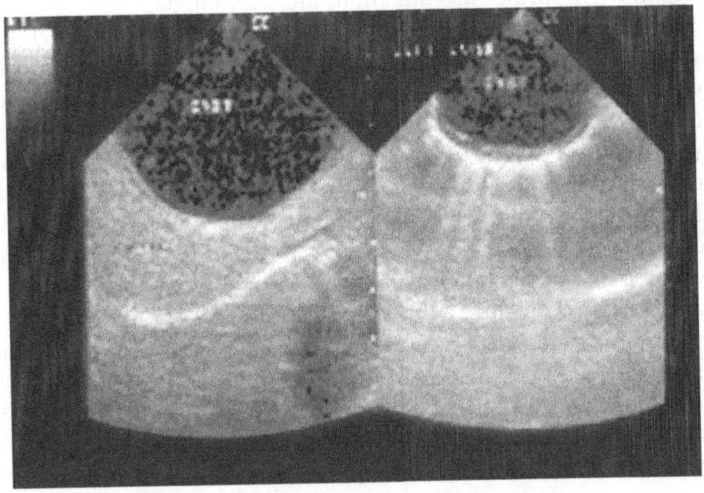

Fig. 26.4: Shows multiple cysts within a large cyst

Lab Investigations

Casoni's test: An intradermal injection of freshly sterilized hydatid fluid gives rise to a large wheal of 5 mm or more size with pseudopodia within half an hour in all positive cases.

Aspiration cytology of the cyst reveals acid-fast hooklets in the aspirate with trichrome stain. However, aspiration is avoided due to fear of spillage of the hydatid fluid causing anaphylaxis.

Urine test may reveal scolices in the urine in renal hydatid cysts.

Blood examination may show high eosinophil count up to 20 to 25%.

Serological and immunological tests are particularly helpful in the diagnosis of coronary and renal involvement. However, with the advantage of the imaging techniques it has its importance only to support the diagnosis.

MANAGEMENT

Surgery

Surgery is the treatment of choice for hepatic hydatid cyst cases and the approach of surgery should be properly selected to get the best result. The procedures usually undertaken are:

1. Cystectomy
2. Pericystectomy
3. PAIR (Puncture, Aspiration, Injection of helminthicides and Reaspiration)
4. Hepatic resection. In selected cases laparoscopic pericystectomy has been well accepted and considered safe and effective when performed in experienced hands.

While performing surgery, care must be taken to prevent spillage of the fluid from the cyst, which causes cyst recurrence. In the surgical procedure, the cyst is sterilized with scolicidal drugs and enucleated. The common scolicidal agents used in the present days are chlorhexidine, hydrogen peroxide, cetrizamide and ethanol. Previously used scolicidals, e.g. hypertonic saline and formalin are not being used at present which can cause fibrosis in the biliary tree.

Indication of hepatic surgery includes large cyst with multiple daughter cysts, a single cyst located superficially with impending danger of spontaneous rupture or rupture due to trauma, infected cyst, cyst causing pressure on adjacent vital organs, cyst communicating into the biliary tract. Cysts communicating to the bilary tract and causing obstruction can be treated by the procedures such as choledochoduodenostomy, endoscopic sphincterotomy and T-tube drainage, etc. Cysts in the brain, spinal cord, kidneys, heart and bone are indicated for surgery. Cysts which are difficult to access or calcified cysts are contraindicated for surgery.

Cysts which cannot be operated can be treated alternatively by PAIR and chemotherapy. There are several cases reported which are accidentally diagnosed by the imageologists while screening for other disease. Some cases may remain asymptomatic for several years. Thus, in some inoperable conditions cases are to be followed-up at intervals.

Chemotherapy

Benzimidazole (Albendazole and mebendazole) is drug of choice for the treatment of Hydatid cysts in case of preoperative and nonoperative conditions. It acts more as parasitostatic drug than parasiticidal. When given after a fatty meal the absorption is better. The efficacy of albendazole is slightly better than mebendazole and is relatively less toxic. Albendazole is given as 400 mg of daily dose for four weeks and repeated with an interval of two weeks for prolonged periods. However, more recently it has been observed that continuous therapy is more efficacious than interrupted therapy. Prolonged therapy with these chemotherapeutics is mandatory, as short-term therapy is insufficient. A combination therapy with praziquintel is considered better than monotherapy in extrahepatic especially bone cysts. However, relapse rates are high with all chemotherapeutic agents.

Prognosis

Successful surgery with complete enucleation of the cyst without spillage gives good result with less chance of recurrence. Pretreatment with benzimidazole prior to surgery shows better prognostic value. The result of treatment of extra hepatic cysts is same as that of hepatic cysts. However, complicated cysts show more chance of mortality.

CONTROL AND PREVENTION

- Personal hygiene like cleaning hands properly before eating.
- Proper cleaning of fruits and green vegetables (green salads) before eating.
- Proper cooking (boiling) of meat.
- Deworming of dogs in endemic areas with proper anthelmintics.
- Laboratory workers and veterinary doctors should guard against contamination while examining the dog's feces.

CONCLUSION

Hydatidosis although occurs globally is seen commonly in temperate climate and countries where cattle, goat and sheep rearing is common. The disease takes years before becoming symptomatic and when diagnosed early and treated carefully has good prognosis. Prevention of the disease by proper personal hygiene, deworming of the dogs and general awareness of disease and its mode of transmission, can reduce the mortality and morbidity to a great extent.

BIBLIOGRAPHY

1. Gottstein B, Reichen J. *Echinococcosis*/Hydatidosis. In: Cook GC, Zumla AI (Eds). Mansons Tropical disease. Saunders Elsevier. 22nd edn. 2003.pp.1549-68.
2. Sinha PR, Jaipuria N, Avasthey P. Intracardiac hydatid cyst and sudden death in a child. Int J Cardiol 1995;51:293-5.

27 *Taenia solium* Cysticercosis in Man and Animals

Chapter

SC Parija, D Kumar, PS Sahu

INTRODUCTION

Among the *Taenia* species only three species *(Taenia saginata, Taenia solium and Taiwan taenia or saginata asiatica or Asian taenia)* are of major public health importance. *Taiwan taenia* is a new species first recognised in Taiwan (Fan,1988), which has been discovered to exist in some Asian Countries such as Taiwan, Philippines, Korea and Indonesia. It has been confirmed as subspecies of *Taenia saginata* (Bowles and Mc Manus,1994) and named as *Taenia saginata asiatica* (Fan et al.,1995). Its cysticerci are found in liver of pigs. In India, Dhanalakshmi (2003) for the first time reported this species in pigs from Bangalore. Taeniasis and cysticercosis are posing continuing threat to the wellbeing of people in many countries through their effects on human health. Animal food industries face rejection and condemnation of infected meat. Developing countries like India are worst affected (Kumar and Gaur, 1994).

Taeniasis and cysticercosis caused by *T. solium* are rampant in many parts of the world particularly where pig farming is common. Cysticercosis is a re-emerging zoonotic global disease classified in the List B by OIE. Approximately 50 million, people are infected with the parasite and about 50,000 die of cysticercosis annually (Eddi et al., 2003). Several reports of patients with cysticercosis from many countries in Asia such as India, China, Indonesia, Thailand, Korea, Taiwan, and Nepal are clear-cut indicators of wide prevalence of *T. solium taeniasis* and cysticercosis (Rajshekhar et al., 2003). In Europe, *T. solium taeniasis* and cysticercosis is endemic in Spain and Portugal but it is rare in most other countries (Schantz et al., 1992). Cysticercosis is endemic in West Cameroon and is an emerging infectious disease in Papua (Irian Jaya) and Indonesia (Wandra et al., 2003).

Neurocysticercosis (NCC) has been diagnosed increasingly in the United States, Scandinavia and Norway as a consequence of increased immigration (Garcia et al., 2004). In India, neurocysticercosis is regarded as the second most important cause of intracranial space occupying lesion (ICSOL) following tuberculosis (Mahajan, 1982) and as the most common cause of epilepsy (Sawhney et al., 1996). Cysticercosis is the cause of epilepsy in up to 50% of Indian patients presenting with partial seizures (Rajshekhar et al., 2003).

HISTORY

The adult *T.solium* and its larval stage have been known since ancient time owing to their large size and common occurrence. Hippocrates described the cysticerci from pigs as early as in 4th century BC and Aristarchus in 5th century BC. Aristotle (384–323 BC) described cysticerci in pigs and wrote "Worm ridden" pigs were those in which there was bad meat on ham neck and shoulder. The name "*Cysticercus*" was given by Laennec, a word derived from Greek word 'Kystic' meaning bladder and 'Kercos' signifying tail (Kumar and Gaur, 1994). Rudolph (1808) gave the name *Cysticercus cellulosae* to larval stage of *T.solium* due to great affinity for connective tissue.

EPIDEMIOLOGY

Worldwide Prevalence

Cysticercosis is prevalent in Mexico, Central and South Africa, Central and South America, India and some areas of Far East (Del Brutto and Sotelo, 1988). This disease is prevalent in areas with low socio-economic status and poor hygiene and sanitation. Overall more than two million people are estimated to have adult tapeworm infection and many more are infected with *Cysticercus*.

Neurocysticercosis is a major cause of epilepsy in Bali, Vietnam, Korea and possibly China and Nepal with rates ranging from 0.02 to 12.6% (Rajshekar et al., 2003). The rates of taeniasis have also been reported to range between 0.1 and 6% in India, Vietnam, China and Bali (Indonesia). An extremely high rate of taeniasis (50%) was reported from an area of Nepal populated by pig rearing farmers (Vedantam et al., 2003). Surveys for human taeniasis in Central and Northern provinces of Hanoi indicated a prevalence of 0.2 to 7.2%. In addition to *T.solium*, *T.saginata* and *T. asiatica* are also known to be present in Vietnam (Willingham et al., 2003).

Taeniasis and cysticercosis have been investigated in detail in Cameroon (Africa) and cysticercosis is a major cause (44.6%) of epilepsy and is present in 0.4 to 3% of the local population (Nguekam et al., 2003). Ophthalmic cysticercosis has been reported from Korea, Mexico, Thailand, Zimbabwe and Canada.

Porcine cysticercosis has been recorded from Africa (Nigeria, West Cameroon), Europe (Poland and Germany), Central and South America (Costa Rica, El salvador, Guatemala, Honduras, Nicaragua, Mexico, Brazil, Chile and Peru) China, Korea and South East Asia (Kumar and Gaur 1994).

Prevalence in India

Neurocysticercosis has been reported from New Delhi, Lucknow, Chennai, Vellore, Chandigarh, Kolkata, Varanasi, Hyderabad, Pondicherry, Bangalore, Mumbai and Ludhiana. Ocular cysticercosis has been recorded from Pondicherry, Chennai, New Delhi, Hyderabad, Chandigarh, Vellore, Aligarh, Rohtak, Mumbai and Ranchi (Parija, 2004). Cysticercosis antibodies or antigen were detected in 6.48% of the healthy blood donors in Pondicherry (Parija et al., 2005).

Ocular cysticercosis has been reported from Pondicherry (Veliath et al., 1985), Delhi (Bajaj and Pushkar, 2002; Verma et al., 2002), Chennai (Sharma et al., 2005), Hyderabad, Chandigarh, Aligarh and Mumbai. The cases of ocular cysticercosis have been reported from Pondicherry (Kaliaperumal et al., 2005; Sahu, 2005).

T. solium cysticercosis in pigs is present in all parts of India but published information is available from a few places. The prevalence varies from place to place which might be due to variation in feeding habits and managemental conditions of that place. The prevalence of porcine cysticercosis from Tamil Nadu, West Bengal, Uttar Pradesh, Bihar, North Eastern region, Andhra Pradesh, Karnataka and Punjab was 7.6%, 4.24%, 5.35 to 15.5%, 7.14%, 20.8 to 36.7%, 4.5%, 6% and 1.75 to 6.35%, respectively. The highest incidence was recorded in North Eastern region followed by Uttar Pradesh (reviewed by Kumar and Gaur, 1994 and D' Souza and Dhanalakshmi, 2005). *T.solium* cysticercosis in pigs is present in Pondicherry but no published information is available.

Economic Impact

The financial losses due to human cysticercosis are very difficult to estimate. The average cost of hospitalization for seizures in one study was Rs. 1615 per patient not including the physician charges (Dias et al., 1999). During course of development the metacestodes migrate through vital organs of the body, including liver and heart before finally attaching the muscle causing severe damage. This may severely affect the quality of carcass causing economic losses to the meat industry. Garrick (1967) estimated a loss of more than $ 500,000 in six Latin American countries due to porcine cysticercosis. No systematic study has been carried out to evaluate the economic implications of cysticercosis in India. A loss of 64,600 rupees due to 3.8% infection in pigs (Pathak and Gaur, 1990a) and 2,61,661 out of 61, 86102 rupees due to 4.22% infection in an organized abattoir in Andhra Pradesh (D'Souza and Hafeez, 1998) has been reported.

Life Cycle

Adult tapeworm is found in the small intestine of man and measures two to six meters and rarely up to 8 meters. Its life cycle completes between man and pig. Pig acts as intermediate host and harbors the larval stage (metacestode/*Cysticercus cellulosae*) and man acts as definitive host harboring adult tapeworm as well as intermediate host harboring the cysticerci. Infection in pigs is usually by direct ingestion of ova. A pig may acquire a heavy infection from a single stool. Unhygienic human behavior is a major factor in transmission of infection. Infection is common in areas where villagers are not provided with sanitary facilities and the pigs run loose scavenging for food (Soulsby, 1882). The prevalence of cysticercosis increases with the age of pigs.

The *cysticercus* in the muscle is digested by gastric juice in stomach, which causes the scolex to evaginate. The scolex anchors itself to the wall of the small intestine and develops into asexually mature adult tapeworm within 5 to 12 weeks. The gravid proglottides full of eggs are passed in chain of five to six and are infective to pig and also to man. The youngest cysticerci are infrequently found in the abdominal cavity between 24 to 72 hours after infection. The lingual, masseter, diaphragmatic and cardiac muscles are mainly affected but liver, kidneys, lungs, brain, heart and eye may also be involved (Kumar and Gaur,1994). The cysticerci may require about ten weeks for complete development in pigs. The lifecycle is completed when man eats raw or semi or undercooked infected 'measly pork'. Heart of the pig naturally infected with *Cysticercus cellulosae* has been shown in the **(Fig. 27.1)**.

Man acquires taeniasis on ingestion of raw or inadequately cooked pork harboring the cysticerci, and by ingestion of food and water contaminated by the eggs particularly if improperly washed vegetable are eaten as salad. Endogenous autoinfection may occur with poor personal hygiene. Autoinfection by reverse peristalsis of intestine once considered to be important is now largely discounted as a source of human infection.

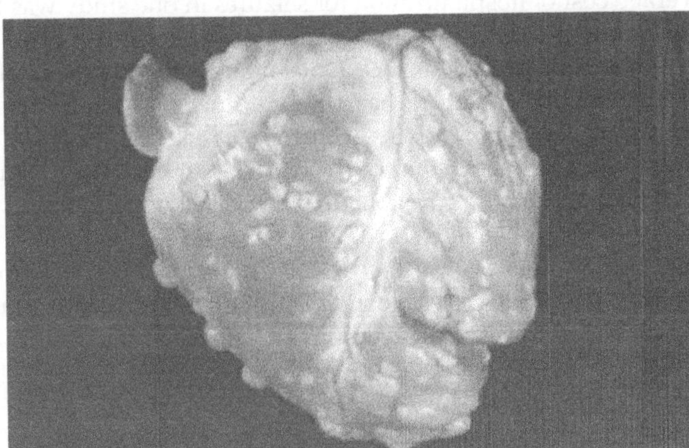

Fig. 27.1: Heart of the pig naturally infected with *Cysticercus cellulosae*

Symptoms

Man

Cysticercosis is the most important clinical manifestation of *T. solium* infection in man, caused by the larval stage/metacestode (*Cysticercus cellulosae*) of the parasite. The clinical symptoms caused by *cysticercus* depend upon the number, size and location of the cysticerci, host immune responses and sequelae of previous infection. The cysticercosis may be classified broadly into asymptomatic and symptomatic groups. Cysticerci have predilection for the central nervous system (CNS), eye and subcutaneous tissue. When cysticerci develop in brain and spinal cord of the central nervous system, the condition is called as neurocysticercosis (NCC), similarly that of eye is called as ocular or extraocular cysticercosis depending upon the location of the cysticerci.

Neurocysticercosis: It is the most serious clinical manifestation of cysticercosis that depends on the number, size and location of cysticerci in CNS. Among the symptoms, recurrent seizures are most common. Other clinical symptoms are raised intracranial pressure, chronic meningitis, abnormal psychiatric manifestations, encephalitis and radiculomyelopathy due to involvement of the spinal cord and its covering membranes. The frequency of seizures can be as high as 91.8%. The seizures may be generalized or local and the focus identified by visual or olfactory hallucinations, amnesia and other varieties of aura (McCormick et al., 1982). CT or MRI increasingly reveals the mimicking idiopathic epilepsy. Raised intracranial pressure is associated with headache, vomiting and papilledema with or without focal neurological sign. Progressive loss of intellect and memory, change in behavior, confusion and disorientation are common psychiatric signs, which may be seen in up to 5% of patients (Mahajan et al., 2004). Focal signs are more commonly seen in the patient in whom cerebral hemisphere involvement is more than the hindbrain. In such cases hemiparesis, dysphasia, visual disturbance and cognitive impairments are more frequently detected. Paraplegia and other signs are seen in spinal cord involvement due to extra or intramedullary compression (Mathuriya et al., 2001). Headache, vertigo, vomiting, papilledema, an altered level of consciousness and gait disturbances may be present in patients with meningeal cysticercosis (Sotelo et al., 1985)

Ophthalmic Cysticercosis: The subretinal space is considered to be the most common site of intraocular cysticercosis (Bartholomew,1975) and 91% of the cysts have been localized in this space or vitreous (Topilow et al., 1981). Intravitreous or subretinal cysts usually lead to blindness within three to five years unless the parasite is surgically removed from the eye. Ocular cysticercosis is commonly seen in Indian subcontinent and sub-conjunctival space is more common site (Malik et al., 1968).

Ocular cysticercosis is initially asymptomatic but in later stages symptoms are due to increase in cyst size or destruction of eyeball by the chronic inflammatory reaction. Wide varieties of manifestations are seen in ocular cysticercosis. They are localized edema, pain, blepharitis, blepharoptosis, conjunctivitis, sub-conjunctival abscess, extraocular muscle myositis, restricted ocular motility, proptosis, uveitis, optic atrophy, papilledema, retinal breaks, chorioretinal exudative or hematogeous retinal detachment (Cano, 2001 and Sharma et al., 2003). The clinical manifestations of orbital or adnexal cysticercosis are entirely different and depend on the location, size, relation to adjacent structures and stage of evolution of the cyst. *Cysticercus cellulosae* cyst in the conjunctiva has been shown in **(Fig. 27.2)**.

Cysticercosis of Muscle: Cysticerci in the muscles are usually silent but a massive pseudohypertrophy of muscle simulating myopathy has been reported. Soft palpable subcuticular nodules are observed on clinical examinations.

Oral Cysticercosis: Oral cysticercosis may occur occasionally and a total of 26 cases have been reported so far. A confirmed case has been reported in an Indian male with nodules in the tongue, lower lip and subcutaneous tissues.

Pig

Clinical symptoms of *T. solium* cysticercosis in pigs are usually absent and the animals appear to be perfectly healthy despite their heavy infection. Noticeable clinical manifestations are found in those cases in which

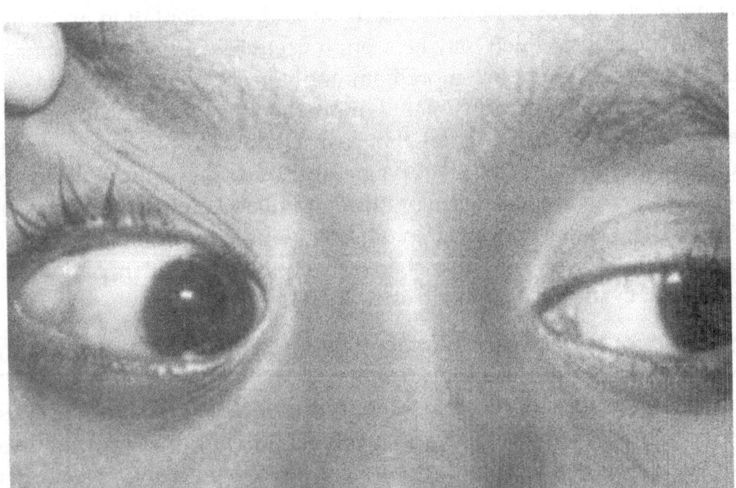

Fig. 27.2: Ophthalmic cysticercosis in human. *Cysticercus cellulosae* in the conjunctiva

cysticerci get lodged in the eye and brain. However, different clinical manifestations are circular movement, epileptic convulsions with grinding of teeth, profuse salivation, unsteady gait, blindness, symptoms similar to rabies, encephalitis, paralysis of tongue, inability to retain food, increased snout sensitivity, general weakness, depression, acute myositis, excitement and diarrhea and death (Kumar and Gaur, 1994).

Diagnosis

Man

Cysticercosis is conventionally diagnosed by palpation biopsy and radiological examination of dead and calcified cysts. But live cysts (noncalcified) are difficult to be seen on X-ray image. The diagnosis should be supported by other tests such as electroencephalogram (EEG), computed tomography (CT) and magnetic resonance imaging (MRI), which confirm the presence of different space occupying lesions in various sites. The immunodiagnostic tests are useful for the demonstration of anticysticercus antibodies and antigen of the parasite.

Neurocysticercosis (NCC): The modern imaging methods (CT and MRI) have greatly improved the accuracy of the diagnosis of NCC by providing evidence on the number and topography of lesions, their stage of involution and the degree of inflammatory reaction of the host against the parasites (Garcia and Del Brutto, 2005).

CT scan is very useful for cysticercosis encephalitis but is less useful for intraventricular or subarachnoid cysts, which can be detected by MRI. The contrast CT scan of brain showing an active cyst with minimal enhancing wall and eccentrically located hyperattenuated nodule suggestive of scolex has been shown in the **(Fig. 27.3)**.

Immunodiagnosis: Immunological tests are being increasingly used in adjunct with imaging techniques to aid the diagnosis of NCC. Immunodiagnostic techniques include detection methods for specific antibodies and for circulating parasite antigen in the serum and CSF (Parija, 2004).

Demonstration of specific antibody in serum and CSF by EITB or ELISA continues to be the mainstay in serodiagnosis of cysticercosis. The EITB using purified *T.solium* glycoprotein antigens is used as the immunodiagnostic test of choice and is recommended in routine diagnosis of cysticercosis by WHO and the Pan American Health Organization (PAHO) (Aguilar-Rebolledo et al., 2002). However, complexity and difficulties in clinical and epidemiological application of the EITB in developing countries is the noted limitation of the test (Carpio, 1999). Evaluations of several commercially available ELISA kits are also reported to be of poor specificity (Hira et al., 2004).

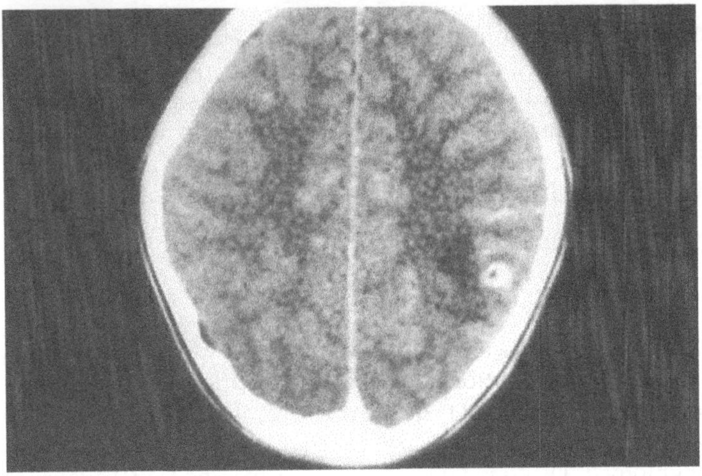

Fig. 27.3: Contrast enhanced CT scan of human brain showing an active cyst with minimal enhancing wall and eccentrically located hyperattenuated nodule suggestive of scolex

The antibody detection has an important drawback in clinical settings: it may indicate exposure to infection and not necessarily the presence of a viable infection, because the serum antibodies may persist long after the parasite has been eliminated by immune mechanisms and/or drug therapy (Garcia et al., 2001). Hence, detection of parasite specific antigens in the serum or CSF is a useful marker in the diagnosis and prognosis of cysticercosis (Pardini et al., 2001) and in the seroepidemiological studies of NCC in endemic areas (Parija et al., 2005).

Antigen detection is preferred because it can distinguish between recent and past infections and can be used to monitor the progress of the therapy.

Of late, use of non-blood specimens such as urine, saliva and tear, which can be collected easily by non-invasive method, is being practised for diagnosis of cysticercosis. Parija et al., (2004) for the first time demonstrated urinary cysticercal antigen in the diagnosis of NCC. Sahu (2005) diagnosed human cysticercosis by antigen detection in urine and tears. Higher specificity and a lower sensitivity of specific immunoglobulin response have been observed in saliva in comparison to serum (Bueno et al., 2000). Malla and Mahajan (2001) recommended the antibody ELISA use for routine diagnosis and epidemiology of NCC.

Pigs

The diagnosis of porcine cysticercosis by examining the tongue to detect the presence of cysticerci is a method known since 379 AD. Cysticerci situated under the lingual mucosa can be easily seen in the form of transparent cyst but parasitic nodules situated deep in the tongue has to be detected by palpation. Tongue examination has been found to be fairly sensitive (70%) and highly specific (100%) and can be used for epidemiologic surveys (Gonzalez et al., 1990). Conventional meat inspection for the diagnosis of *T.solium* cysticercosis in pigs often fails to detect mild cases of infection (Kumar and Gaur, 1994).

The serological diagnosis of porcine cysticercosis is a difficult task due to marked cross reactivity between infection with one taeniid metacestode and another. The modern technique of CT is of great importance for humans but its application to animal infection in field conditions is questionable due to economic implications particularly in developing countries (Kumar and Gaur, 1994).

Various workers have tried various serological tests (DID, IEP, CIEP, ELISA, EITB) with variable results depending upon the type of antigens. Since the quality of antigen used to play a major role in the specificity and sensitivity of an immunodiagnostic tests, stress has been placed on fractionation and characterization of antigens (Kumar et al., 1987a). Although immunodiffusion test is simpler and does not require any sophisticated equipment or reagent, it has poor sensitivity. The IHA has been found to be highly sensitive with different types necessary to achieve the optimum sensitivity and specificity (Kumar and Gaur, 1990a). IEP is quite specific and economical but lacks the desired level of sensitivity (Kumar and Gaur, 1989c).

Kumar and Gaur (1989) compared the sensitivity of DID, IHA, IEP, CIEP and ELISA. Highest sensitivity was obtained with ELISA and lowest with DID. Latex agglutination test has been found as efficient as ELISA (Prasanna et al., 2001). D'Souza and Hafeez (1999a and b) and Dhanalakshmi (2003) observed that E-5 antigen proved to be best. Enzyme immuno transfer blot (EITB) has been considered as valuable method for the diagnosis of porcine cysticercosis (Sreenivasamurthy et al., 1999 and Dhanalakshmi, 2003). Dhanalakshmi et al., (2006) have standardized Protein-A ELISA for the diagnosis of porcine cysticercosis.

Several PCR based assays for detection of *T.solium* eggs, proglottids and larval stage from human and pig tissue have been described. Preliminary evaluation has shown these assays to be reliable, sensitive and specific (Meri and Mere, 2002).

Treatment

The control and eradication of taeniasis and cysticercosis in man and animals is very difficult because of local habits, traditions and practices of people in cooking, food management and feeding of domestic animals and religious ceremonies (Kumar and Gaur, 1994).

Earlier extract of male fern, kamala betel nuts and a paste from pumpkin seed were used for the treatment of adult tapeworm. However, with the production of new effective anthelmintics the use of these medicines decreased. A safe and effective treatment of intestinal tapeworm infection may be achieved with either praziquantel or niclosamide, the well tolerated oral agents that have direct cysticidal effect (Carpio et al., 2002).

Now-a-days praziquantel at a dosage of 10 mg/kg is considered as drug of choice for adult tapeworm *Taenia* spp. (White and Weller, 2008). However, single dose may aggravate central nervous system (CNS) inflammation, if there is a cryptic CNS lesion. Niclosamide (2 g single dose) is other safe and effective drug. Its administration should be followed by a mild laxative after one to two hours to prevent retrograde intestinal autoinfection. Albendazole (400–800 mg) has 85% efficacy.

Several drugs including fenbendazole, praziquantel, albendazole and oxfendazole have been used as chemotherapeutic agents in experimental and natural porcine cysticercosis. Albendazole and praziquantel have a major limitation since these drugs have to be administered over several days. Oxfendazole, however, has the advantage that it can be administered in single dose (30 mg/kg). The drug causes complete disappearance of cysts at 12 weeks after treatment and pork is rendered clean with no residual cyst or scar thereby increasing the value in pork market (Gonzalez, 2002).

Treatment of NCC

Therapeutic measures in human NCC include antiparasitic drugs, surgery and symptomatic treatment. Prior to the advent of antiparasitic drugs, surgery was the primary therapy for excision of large cysts or cysts in the ventricles. The role of surgical therapy in the management of NCC has significantly decreased over time and is mainly restricted to placement of ventricular shunts for hydrocephalus secondary to NCC.

Although albendazole and praziquantel are effective antiparasitic drugs against the cysticerci, the treatment of NCC still remains controversial (Singhal and Salines, 2002).

Praziquantel at an oral dose of 50 to 60 mg per kg daily in three divided doses for 15 to 30 days (or at least for 10 days) is recommended (White and Weller, 2008; Todd et al., 2006). A single day regimen of praziquantel has recently been described with similar rate of cyst disappearance in some patients (Del Brutto et al., 1999).

Albendazole at the dose of 15 mg per kg per day for one month was initially recommended, but a shorter course of the same daily dose for seven to eight days has become the treatment of choice now (Sotelo et al., 1988; Todd et al., 2006). Albendazole is less expensive and has better penetration ability into cerebrospinal fluid.

Both agents may exacerbate inflammatory response around dying parasite, thereby exacerbating seizures or hydrocephalus. Thus, high dose corticosteroids and antiepileptic drugs should be used during treatment period.

In patients with diffuse cerebral edema and raised intracranial pressure due to multiple inflamed lesions, glucocorticoids are the mainstay of treatment and antiparasitic drugs should be avoided (White and Weller, 2008).

Treatment of Ophthalmic Cysticercosis

A combination of oral albendazole and corticosteroids is found to be effective in cases of ophthalmic cysticercosis (Kaliaperumal et al., 2005). However, drug induced inflammation may cause irreversible damage; thus, most patients should be managed surgically (White and Weller, 2008).

Vaccination

Porcine cysticercosis can be controlled either by mass anthelmintic treatment or with an effective vaccine. Partial protection has been achieved by vaccination of healthy pigs with crude and fractionated antigen of scolices (Kumar et al., 1987b), extract of egg antigen (Kumar and Gaur, 1990b), antigen from *in-vitro* culture of onchospheres (Pathak and Gaur, 1990b) and *T. solium* onchospheres antigens (Verastegui et al., 2003). The recombinant onchospheres antigens (TSOL 18 and TSOL45-1A) have provided 100% protection and could be basis for development of highly effective vaccine that could control and eradicate the human NCC (Lightowlers, 2003 and Flessar et al., 2004).

Control

Control and eradiction of cysticercosis is a diffcult task because of local habits, traditions and practices (Kumar and Gaur, 1994). However, it could be possible by involving medical, public health and veterinary professionals along with mass education of people. The proper disposal of human excreta, restriction on scavenging habit of pigs, careful meat inspection and avoiding contamination of vegetable by human stool/feces can reduce the incidence of infection. Eating of raw or undercooked pork should be avoided. Prompt treatment of infected people will not only reduce the source of infection, but will also eliminate the danger of autoinfection with cysticerci. Though cooking of pork is the most effective means of prophylaxis, cysticerci are killed by heating at 45 to 55°C but pork should be cooked for at least one and half hours for every pound, or until it becomes grey in color. Freezing below –20°C also kills cysticerci but at 0 to 2°C they survive for nearly two months and at room temperature for 26 days. Freezing at –10°C for four or more days is an effective but expensive procedure. Pickling is not always successful. *T. solium* cysticerci are more resistant to acid than basic solutions. Keeping in view the gravity of the problem, the FAO through the Veterinary Public Health and Food Safety Program is in process of establishing regional networks located in Asia, Africa, Eastern and Central Europe and Latin America which will provide a basic framework to spread information (Eddi et al., 2003).

CONCLUSION

Eradication of *T.solium* cysticercosis is difficult but not impossible, if combined efforts are made for the treatment of human taeniasis and porcine cysticercosis. With the advancement of molecular parasitology, the development of suitable diagnostic kit and effective recombinant vaccine (against *T.solium* cysticercosis) are possible. Above all, public health education of people will be of great help to achieve the goal of eradication.

BIBLIOGRAPHY

1. Aguilar-Rebolledo F, Meza-Lucas A, Torres J, Cedillo-Rivera R, Enciso A, Garcia RC, Munoz O, Correa D. Evaluation of the enzyme-linked immunoelectrotransfer blot assay for diagnosis of neurocysticercosis in children. J Child Neurol 2002;17(6):416-20.
2. Bajaj MS, Pushker N. Optic nerve cysticercosis. Clin Experiment Ophthalmol 2002;30:140-3.
3. Bartholomew RS, Subretinal cysticercosis. Am J Ophthalmol 1995;79:670-3.
4. Bowles J, Mc Manus DP. Genetic characterization of the Asian, a Taenia, newly described taeniid cestode of human. Am J Trop Med Hyg 1994;50:33-44.
5. Bueno EC, Vaz AJ, Machado LD, Livramento JA. Neurocysticercosis: detection of IgG, IgA and IgE antibodies in cerebrospinal fluid, serum and saliva samples by ELISA with *Taenia solium* and *Taenia crassiceps* antigens. Arq Neuropsiquiatr 2000;58:18-24.
6. Cano MR Ocular cysticercosis. In: Retina Stephen J Ryan. 3rd edn. Mosby: 2001;2;1553-7..
7. Carpio A Diagnostic criteria for human cysticercosis. J Neurol Sci 1998;161: 185-8.
8. Carpio A, Hauser WA. Prognosis for seizure recurrence in patients with newly diagnosed neurocysticercosis Neurology 2002;59:1730-34.
9. Del Brutto OH, Sotelo J. Neurocysticercosis: An update Rev Infec Dis 1998;10:1075-87.
10. Del Brutto OH, Campos X, Sanchez J, Mosquera A. Single-day praziquantel versus 1-week albendazole for neurocysticercosis Neurology 1999;52:1079-81.
11. Dhanalakshmi H. PhD thesis entitled "Phenotypic and genotypic characterization and imunodiagnosis of *Taenia solium* bladder worms of pigs" submitted to University of Agricultural Sciences, Bangalore 2003.
12. Dhanalakshmi H, Jagannath MS, Isloor S, D'Souza PE. Protein-A ELISA in the diagnosis of porcine cysticercosis J Vet Parasitol 2006;20:33-5.
13. D'Souza PE, Hafeez Md. Incidence of *Cysticercus cellulosae* infection in pigs in Andhra Pradesh, Mysore. J Agri Sci 1998;32(1):75-8.
14. D'Souza PE, Hafeez Md. Detection of *Taenia solium* cysticercosis in pigs by ELISA with an Excretory Secretory antigen. Vet Res Commn 1999a;23:293-8.
15. D'Souza PE, Hafeez Md. Comparison of routine meat inspection, CIEP and ELISA to detect *Cysticercus cellulosae* infection in pigs. Indian Vet J 1999b;76: 285-8.
16. D'Souza PE, Dhanalakshmi H. Cysticercosis in pigs-Epidemiology, immunodiagnosis, economic impact under Indian conditions and control. Intal Polivet (vet Parasitol Spl Issue) 2005;6:229-96.

17. Eddi C, Nari A, Amanfu W. *Taenia solium* cysticercosis/taeniasis: potential linkage with FAO activities: FAO support possibilities Acta Tropica 2003;87:145-8.
18. Fan PC. *Taiwan Taenia* and taeniasis Parasitol Today 1988;4:86-8.
19. Fan PC, Lin CY, Chen CC, Chung WC. Morphological description of *Taenia saginata asiatica* from man in Asia. J Helminthol 1995;69:299-303.
20. Flisser A, Gauci CG, Zoli A, Martinez-Ocana J, Garza-Rodriguez A, Dominguez Alpizar JL, et al. Induction of protection against porcine cysticercosis by vaccination with recombinant oncosphere antigens. Infect Immun 2004;72(9):5292-7.
21. Garcia HH, Del Brutto OH. Cysticercosis Working Group in Peru. Neurocysticercosis: updated concepts about an old disease. Lancet Neurol 2005;4:653-61.
22. Garcia HH, Gonzalez AE, Gilman RH, Palacios LG, Jimenez I, Rodriguez S, Verastegui M, Wilkins P, Tsang VC. Cysticercosis Working Group in Peru. Short report: transient antibody response in *Taenia solium* infection in field conditions-a major contributor to high seroprevalence. Am J Trop Med Hyg 2001;65(1):31-2.
23. Garcia HH, Pretell EJ, Gibman RH, Martinez SM, Moulton LH, Del Brutto OH, Herrer G, Evans CA, Gonzalez AE. Cysticercosis Working Group in Peru. A trial of antiparasitic treatment to reduce the rate of seizures due to cerebral cysticercosis. N Engl J Med 2004;350:249-58.
24. Garrick D. Estado actual delabrucelosis, tuberculosis rabia y cicticercosis en centroamerica y Panama. Boletin de la oficina santaria Panamericana 1967;63:142-50.
25. Gonzalez AE. Control of *Taenia solium* with porcine chemotherapy. In: *Taenia solium* cysticercosis from Basic to Clinical Science. Singh G. Prabhakarss (Eds). CABI Publishing, CAB International, Willingford, RK 2002.pp.431-5.
26. Gonzalez AE, Cama V, Gilman RH. Prevalence and comparison of serological assay, necropsy and tongue examination for the diagnosis of porcine cysticercosis in Peru. Am J Trop Med Hyg 1990;43:194-9.
27. Hira PR, Francis I, Abdella NA, Gupta R, Ai-Ali FM, Grover S, Khalid N, Abdeen S, Iqbal J, Wilson M, Tsang VC. Cysticercosis: imported and autochthonous infections in Kuwait. Trans R Soc Trop Med Hyg 2004;98 (4):233-9.
28. Kaliaperumal S, Rao VA, Parija SC. Cysticercosis of the eye in South India-a case series Indian J Med Microbiol 2005;23:227-30.
29. Kumar D, Gaur SNS. Counterimmunoelectrophoresis in the diagnosis of *Taenia solium* cysticercosis in pigs using fractionated antigens. J Vet Parasitol 1987a;1:43-6.
30. Kumar D, Gaur SNS. Serodiagnosis of porcine cysticercosis by enzyme linked immunosorbent assay (ELISA) using fractionated antigens. Vet Parasitol 1987b;24:195-202.
31. Kumar D, Gaur SNS. Comparative evaluation of various immunodiagnostic tests for the diagnosis of *Taenia solium* cysticercosis in pig using fractionated antigens. J Helm 1989;63:13-7.
32. Kumar D, Gaur SNS. Complement fixation test in the diagnosis of *Taenia solium* cystecercosis in pigs using scolex antigen. Indian J Vet Med 1990a;10:71-3.
33. Kumar D, Gaur SNS. Immunisation of piglets against cysticercus of *Taenia solium* using an extract of *Taenia solium* eggs. Indian J Comp Micro Imun and Infect Dis 1990b;11:44-5.

34. Kumar D, Gaur SNS. *Taenia solium* cysticercosis in pigs. Helminthological Abstracts, CAB International, UK 1994;63:365-83.
35. Kumar D, Gaur SNS, Pathak KML. Fractionation and characterization of cysticercus of *Taenia solium*. Res Vet Sci 1987a;43:395-7.
36. Kumar D, Gaur SNS, Pathak KML. Immunization of pigs against cysticercus of *Taenia solium*, using fractioned 1st and 2nd peaks of Cysticercus cellulosae scolex antigen. Indian J Ani Sci 1987b;57:932-5.
37. Kumar D, Gaur SNS, Varshney KC. Indirect fluorescent antibody test in the diagnosis of porcine cysticercosis. Indian J Ani Sci 1987c;57:1204-6.
38. Lightowlers WW. Vaccines for prevention of cysticercosis. Acta Tripica 2003;87:129-35.
39. Mahajan RC. Geographical distribution of human cysticercosis. In: Cysticercosis: Present state of knowledge and prospective. Flisser A, Williams K, Laclette JP, Larralde C, Ridaura C, Beltran F (Eds). Academic Press Inc. New York 11982;39-46.
40. Mahajan K, Machhan PC, Sood BR, Kumar S, Sharma DP, Mokta J, Pal LS. Neurocysticercosis presenting with psychosis. J Assoc Physician India 2004;52:663-5.
41. Malla N, Mahajan RC. Human neurocysticercosis. In: Sood ML (Ed). Helminthology in India. International Bood Distributors, Dehradun (India) 2001.pp.247-62.
42. Malik SR, Gupta AK, Choudhry S. Ocular cysticercosis. Am J Ophthalamol 1968;66:1168-71.
43. Mathuriya SN, Khosla VK, Vasishta RK, Tewari MK, Pathak A, Prabhakar S. Intramedullary cysticercosis: MRI diagnosis. Neuro India 2001;49:71-4.
44. Meri T, Meri S. Polymerase chain reaction in the diagnosis of *Taenia solium* cysticercosis. In: *Taenia solium* cysticercosis from Basic to Clinical Science. Singh G, Prabhakar S. CABI Publishing, CAB International, Willingford, UK 2002.pp.351-6.
45. Mc Cormick GF, Zee CS, Heiden J Cysticercosis cerebri. Review of 127 cases Arch Neurol 1982;39:534-9.
46. Nguekam JP, Zoli AP, Zogo PO, Kamga AC, Speybroeck N, Dorny P, Brandt J, Lesson B, Geerts SA. Seroepidemiological study of human cysticercosis in West Cameroon. Trop Med Int Health 2003;8:144-9.
47. Pardini AX, Vaz AJ, Dos Ramos Machado L, Livramento JA. Cysticercus antigens in cerebrospinal fluid samples from patients with neurocysticercosis. J Clin Microbiol 2001;39(9):3368-72.
48. Parija SC. Text Book of Medical Parasitology. 2nd edn. All India Publishers and Distributors Chennai India; 2004.
49. Parija SC, Balamurugan N, Sahu PS, Subbaiah SP, Cysticercus antibodies and antigen in serum from blood donors from Pondicherry India Rev Inst Med Trop Sao Paulo 2005;47:227-0.
50. Parija M, Biswas R, Harish BN, Parija SC. Detection of specific cysticercus antigen in urine for the diagnosis of neurocysticercosis. Acta Trop 2004;92:253-60.
51. Parija SC, Sahu PS. A serological study of human cysticercosis in Pondicherry, South India. J Commun Dis 2003;35:283-9.
52. Parija SC, Sahu PS. Evaluation of human 'O' positive blood cells (RBCs) stabilized with various aldehydes in the indirect hemagglutination (IHA) test for diagnosis of neurocysticercosis. J Parasit Dis 2004a;28:96-101.

53. Parija SC, Sahu PS. Evaluation of chick red blood cells stabilized with various aldehydes in the indirect hemagglutination (IHA) test for diagnosis of neurocysticercosis. J Vet Parasit 2004b;19:9-14.
54. Pathak KML, Gaur SNS. Prevalence and economic implications of *Taenia solium* taeniasis and cysticercosis in Uttar Pradesh state of India. Acta Leidensia 1990a;57:197-200.
55. Pathak KML, Gaur SNS. Immunization of pigs with culture antigens of *Taenia solium*. Vet Parasitol 1990b;34:353-6.
56. Prasanna KM, Jagannath MS, D'Souza PE. Diagnosis of *Taenia solium* cysticercosis in pigs by Latex Agglutination test. J Vet Parasitol 2001;15:47-9.
57. Rajshekhar V, Joshi DD, Doanh NQ, Van De N, Xiaonong Z. *Taenia solium* Taeniasis/cysticercosis in Asia: Epidemiology, impact and issues Acta Trop 2003;87:5360.
58. Sahu PS. Diagnosis of human cysticercosis by antigen detection in urine and tear. Ph.D thesis work carried out at Dept. of Microbiology, JIPMER, Pondicherry and submitted to Pondicherry university Pondicherry. 2005.
59. Sawhney IMS, Lakhra OP, Sashi JS, Prabhakar S, Chopra JS. Evaluation of epilepsy management in a developing country: A prospective study of 407 patients. Acta Neurologica Scandinavica 1996;94:19-3.
60. Selvam P, D'Souza PE, Jagannath MS. Serodiagnosis of *Taenia Solium* cysticercosis in pigs by indirect hemagglutination test. Veterinarski Archiv 2004;74:453-8.
61. Schantz PM, Moore AC, Munoz JL, Hartman BJ, Schaefer JA, Aron AM, Persaud D, Sati E, Wilson M, Flisser A. Neurocysticercosis in an orthodox Jewish Community in New York City. N Engl J Med 1992;327:692-5.
62. Sharma T, Sinha S, Shah N, Gopal L, Shanmugam MP, Bhende P, Bhende M, Shetty NS, Agrawal R, Deshpande D, Biswas J, Sukumar B, Intraocular cysticercosis: Clinical characteristics and visual outcome after Vitroretinal surgery Opthalmol 2003;110:996-1004.
63. Singal BS, Salinas RA. Controversies during treatment of neurocysticercosis. In: *Taenia solium* cysticercosis from Basic to Clinical science. G Singh and S Prabhakar (Eds) CABI Publishing, CAB Internationl, Willingford, UK 2002.pp.421-6.
64. Sreenivasamurthy GS, D'Souza PE, Jagannath MS. Enzyme linked immunoelectrotransfer blot in the diagnosis of *Taenia solium* cysticercosis in pigs J Para Dis 1999;23:85-8.
65. Sotelo J, Torres B, Rubio-Donnadieu F, Escobedo F, Rodriguez-Carbujal J. Praziquantel in the treatment of neurocysticercosis: Long term follow-up Neurology 1985;35:752-5.
66. Sotelo J, Guerrero J, Rubio F. A new classification based on active and inactive forms. Arch Intern Med 1988;148:442-5.
67. Soulsby EJL. In: Helminths, Arthropods and Protozoa of Domesticated Animals 7th edn. ELBS and Bailliere, Tindall and Cassell, London. 1982.
68. Todd WTA, Lockwood DNJ, Sundar S. Infectious diseases In: Boon NA, Colledge NR, Walker BR (Eds). Davidson's Principles and Practice of Medicine. 20th edn. Churchill Livingstone, Edinburgh 2006.pp.283-376.
69. Topilow HW, Yimoyine DJ, Freeman HM, Young GA, Addison R. Bilateral multifocal intraocular cysticercosis. Opthalmol 1981;88:1166-72.
70. Vedantam R, Joshi DD, Nguyen QD, Nguyen-van-De, Zhou-X. *Taenia solium* taeniasis/cysticercosis in Asia: Epidemiology, impact and issues. Acta-Tropica 2003;83:53-60.

71. Veliath AJ, Ratnakar C, Thakur LC, Cysticercosis in South India. J Trop Med Hyg 1985;88:25-9.
72. Verma L, Agrawal T, Kulkarni A, Mahajan H, Tandon R. Optic nerve cysticercosis. Arch Opthalmol 2002;120:1408-9.
73. Verastegui M, Gilman RH, Garcia HH, Gouzalez AE, Arana Y, Jeri C, Tuero I, Gavidia CM, Levine M, Tsang VC. Cysticercosis Working Group in Peru. Prevalence of antibodies to unique *Taenia solium* onchosphere antigens in taeniasis and human and porcine cysticercosis. Am J Trop Med Hyg 2003;69:438-44.
74. Wandra T, Ito A, Yamasaki H, Surozo T, Margono SS, *Taenia solium* cysticercosis, Irian jaya, Indonesia. Emerg Infec Dis 2003;9:884-5.
75. White AC, Weller PF, Cestodes. In: Fauci AS, Braunwald E, Kasper DL, et al. (Eds). Harrison's Principles of Internal Medicine 17th edn. Mc Graw Hill, New York 2008:1336-41.
76. Willingham AL, 3rd De NV, Doanh NQ, Cong Le D, Dung TV, Dorny P, Cam PD, Dalsgard A. Current status of cysticercosis in Vietnam. South-East Asian J Trop Med Pub Health 34(Suppl-1). 2003;35-50.

28 Chapter

Lymphatic Filariasis–Revisited

SP Pani, LK Das

INTRODUCTION

Lymphatic filariasis in humans is caused by lymphatic dwelling nematode parasites: *Wuchereria bancrofti, Brugia malayi and Brugia timori*. In India, *Wuchereria bancrofti* constitutes to 99% and *Brugia malayi* 1%. According to the latest global estimate, India alone contributes to about 41% of the global burden of lymphatic filariasis **(Table 28.1)**. This disease has been identified as the second most important cause of permanent disability and, one of the six diseases, which can be eliminated.

HISTORY OF THE DISEASE

Lymphatic filariasis has been a major public health problem in India next to malaria. This disease was recorded in India as early as 6th century BC by the famous Indian physician Susruta in his book *Susrut Samhita*. In 7th century AD, Madhavakara described the signs and symptoms of the disease in his treatise *Madhava Nidhana* which holds well even today. In 1709, Clarke described elephantoid legs as' 'Malabar legs'. The discovery of the life cycle by Patrick Manson in 1877 is regarded as one of the most significant discoveries in tropical medicine.

Table 28.1: Relative magnitude of problem due to *Wuchereria bancrofti* (Wb) and *Brugia malayi* (Bm), comparison between global and Indian estimates (in millions)

Parameters	*Global*		*India*		*India as % global*	
	Wb	*Bm*	*Wb*	*Bm*	*Wb*	*Bm*
Microfilaria carriers	73.3	10.4	29.5	1.8	40.2	17.3
Lymphedema	13.2	2.8	6.9	0.9	52.3	32.1
Hydrocele	25.8	NA*	12.9	NA*	48.1	NA*
Total #	106.2	12.9	45.5	2.6	42.8	20.2

The total cases exclude a proportion of individuals who may have overlapping infection/ lymphedema/hydrocele.

* Not applicable, since *B. malayi* does not result in hydrocele.

THE PATHOGEN

In India, lymphatic filariasis is caused by two lymphatic dwelling nematode parasites; namely, *Wuchereria bancrofti* and *Brugia malayi*. These parasites exhibit cyclo-developemental life cycle, alternating between human host and vector mosquitoes. The adult parasites inhabit the lymphatics and lymph nodes of man. After mating the oviparous adult female releases microfilaria (larval stage) which reach and circulate in blood exhibiting a nocturnal periodicity. Sub-periodic form of *W. bancrofti* has been reported from the Nicobar island. The microfilaria, when picked-up by susceptible vectors, grows through three larval stages and the third stage larvae are infective to man. This infective L3 grows through two more stages (L4 and L5) to become an adult, which becomes sexually mature in about a year. The fecundic life span (period for which an adult female produces microfilaria) has been estimated to be 5.4 years for *W. bancrofti* and 3.5 years for *B. malayi*. The life span of microfilaria is estimated to be about six months.

THE VECTORS

In India, *W. bancrofti* is transmitted to man by the ubiquitous mosquito, *Culex quinguifaciatus*. This mosquito breeds in polluted water bodies in and around human habitation. This vector is found abundantly in all urban, semi-urban areas, as well as in rural areas, which are undergoing rapid urbanization. In course of time, this vector mosquito has become highly anthropophagic. *B. malayi* in India, is transmitted by *Mansonia* mosquitoes (*M. annulifera, M. uniformis,* and *M. indiana*). These mosquitoes breed in fresh water bodies in association with hydrophytes such as *Pistia, Echornia* and *Salvinia*. Mansonia mosquitoes also show high degree of anthropophilic index. *Aedes (Finlaya) niveus* is the vector of subperiodic *W. bancrofti* in Nicobar islands.

PATHOLOGY AND PATHOGENESIS

The parasite infective larvae, after being dropped from the mouth of the biting vector mosquito on human skin, make their way through the site of the bite (depending upon the micro-climatic conditions) and find their way to the lymph vessels. The parasite moults twice to reach adult stage and after sexual maturity, mate and the female releases microfilaria. The adult parasites result in lymphatic abnormalities such as dilatation, kinking and collateral formation, etc. These changes are initially transiently reversible, but subsequently become permanently irreversible. Despite these changes, in most cases, the pathology remains subclinical for long periods of time. Due to this reason, many parasite carriers remain asymptomatic for years. Depending on the site of the adult parasite localization and the lymphatics involved, the pathogenesis varies. Adult parasites in testicular lymphatics of male (the most preferred site of *W. bancrofti* in this gender) result in passive fluid accumulation between the layers of *tunica* which in turn causes hydrocele, with minimal immunopathology and thus, the microfilaria detection is higher in these cases as compared to in lymphedema fluid. Adult parasites located in deep inguinal or femoral lymphatics in either gender result in gross immunopathology and lymphedema. Lymphedema is initially reversible but slowly becomes irreversible. Large quantity of free fluid remains trapped in lymphatic and tissue spaces until late stages of lymphedema, where fibrosis takes over resulting in solid edema. The skin changes gradually and secondary bacterial infection (particularly due to Group A Beta hemolytic *Streptococcus*) in the protein rich lymph results in repeated attacks of lymphangitis, lymphadenitis and filarial fever (described as acute adeno-lymphangitis (ADL). Repeated attacks of ADL worsen the lymphedema until elephantiasis (roughening and thickening of skin) results. In few cases with *W. bancrofti* infection, a specific hypersensitive response occurs directed against the microfilaria, resulting in an allergic disease with lungs as the target organ which is called as Tropical Pulmonary Eosinophilia.

DIAGNOSIS OF LYMPHATIC FILARIASIS

Traditionally, diagnosis of filarial infections in humans has been by parasitological methods of finding and identifying the prelarval microfilarial (MF) stage of the parasite in human blood. Recently, more often immunological and molecular techniques are being employed. The diagnosis of filarial infection can be now made in following ways:

1. Clinical diagnosis
2. Parasitological diagnosis
3. Ultrasound method of detecting adult worms
4. Immunodiagnosis
5. Molecular diagnosis
6. Detection of parasites in vectors.

Clinical Diagnosis

The major clinical symptoms of lymphatic filariasis (LF) consist of recurrent fever, retrograde lymphangitis, lymphadenitis, orchitis, hydrocele, lymphedema, elephantiasis (advanced form of lymphedema) and minor clinical symptoms consist of tropical pulmonary eosinophilia (TPE), chyluria, monoarticular arthritis and microscopic hematuria. The manifestations can be divided as acute, chronic and other manifestations.

Acute Disease

Fever associated with inflammation of the lymph nodes and/or lymph vessels is termed adenolymphangitis (ADL). In endemic areas, two distinct types of acute ADL are recognized.

i. *AFL:* The first type is acute filarial lymphangitis (AFL), caused by the death of adult worm **(Fig. 28.1)**. AFL has mild clinical symptoms and is a self-limiting condition. In AFL, there is a cord like structure with lymphadenitis and retrograde lymphangitis. The scrotum is commonly involved resulting in funiculo-epididymo-orchitis. Systemic reactions are mild and distal edema is rare.

ii. *ADLA (Figs 28.2 and 28.3):* The second type, most common acute manifestation of the disease is caused by secondary bacterial infections. It is referred to as acute dermato-lymphangio-adenitis (ADLA). It causes severe local and systemic symptoms and does not resolve by itself. The affected limb is warm, tender and painful. In some patients, there is redness of the overlying skin. Lymphadenitis and/or lymphangitis may be present. Constitutional symptoms include high fever, myalgia, headache, chills, nausea, vomiting and giddiness. Both the local and constitutional symptoms severely incapacitate the patient. Fungal infections in web spaces (most of which are asymptomatic) are also frequently observed in these patients which could serve as portal of entry for pathogenic bacteria. Symptoms resolve on treatment with appropriate antibiotics. Progression of lymphedema is enhanced after recurrent attacks of ADLA.

The other forms of acute disease may be as follows:

Acute hydrocele or acute filarial epididymo-orchitis: Acute disease in the male genitalia presents as acute hydrocele or acute epididymo-orchitis. Acute hydrocele is caused by the presence of adult worm in the intrascrotal lymphatics while acute epididymo-orchitis is generally due to secondary bacterial infection. It presents with pain, tenderness and swelling of the scrotum and is usually associated with fever and chills. The testis and epididymis are swollen and tender.

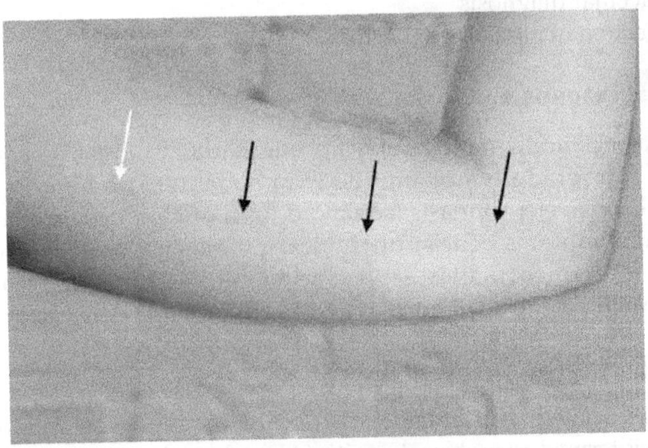

Fig. 28.1: Lymphangitis

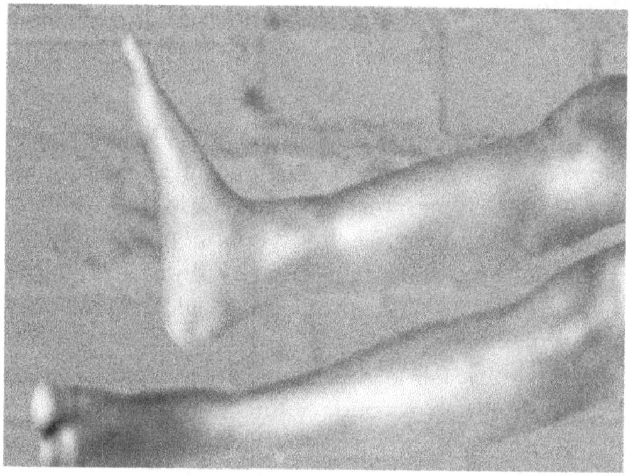

Fig. 28.2: Dermato-lymphangitis of right leg

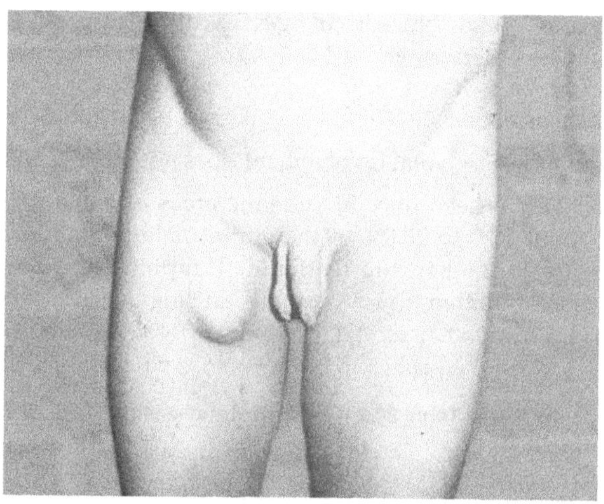

Fig. 28.3: Acute inguinal adenitis

Acute Filarial Chyluria (AFC)

It is a condition with passage of intestinal lymph in urine as "milky urine" in persons residing in areas endemic for lymphatic filariasis. Parasitic infestation damages the intestinal and lumbar lymphatic trunks that drain into cisterna chyli. Generally, patient does not have any symptom except passing milky urine intermittently. Dysuria may be present if there is a clot formation, especially in men. Patient may complain of hemochyluria if it is blood stained.

Chronic Disease

This is seen only in a small proportion of infected individuals.

Involvement of Limbs

Lymphedema (Table 28.2 and Fig. 28.4): Continued and prolonged presence of adult worms in the lymphatics leads to lymph stasis in the affected area and eventually lymphedema. The most common sites of lymphedema are the lower limbs and sometimes upper limbs. Continued lymph stasis results in skin thickening, fibrous tissue proliferation, ulceration, nodule formation and warty growths.

Progressive lymph stasis leads to impairment of lymphatic function and increased susceptibility to secondary infection particularly with bacterial organisms resulting in ADLA which is very distressing to the patient. In brugian filariasis, the lymphedema characteristically affects the limbs below the knee/elbow. Since it is difficult to differentiate lymphedema due to other causes from filarial lymphedema, the current practice is to consider any lymphedema especially unilateral lymphedema (particularly non-pitting and associated with skin changes) in endemic areas as being filarial in origin unless otherwise proved.

Genital Manifestations

In brugian filariasis, genital involvement does not occur.

Hydrocele: This is seen only in endemic areas of bancroftian filariasis affecting about 10.0 to 20.0% of the entire male population. When the parasites are lodged in the testicular lymphatics, it results in the accumulation of fluid in tunica vaginalis causing hydrocele. Hydrocele is differentiated from other scrotal swellings by 'getting over the swelling',

Table 28.2: Grading of lymphedema

Grade of lymphedema	*Edema*	*Reversibility*	*Overlying skin*	*Treatment*
Grade-I	Pitting	Completely reversible on elevation	Normal	Limb elevation
Grade-II	Pitting or nonpitting	Not reversible on elevation	Normal	Limb elevation, pneumatic compression
Grade-III	Non-pitting	Not reversible on elevation	Skin thickened	Limb elevation, pneumatic compression, leg hygiene
Grade-IV	Non-pitting	Not reversible on elevation	Skin thickened, hyperkeratosis, nodules, wart, etc. (elephantiasis).	Limb elevation, leg hygiene, local antibiotics

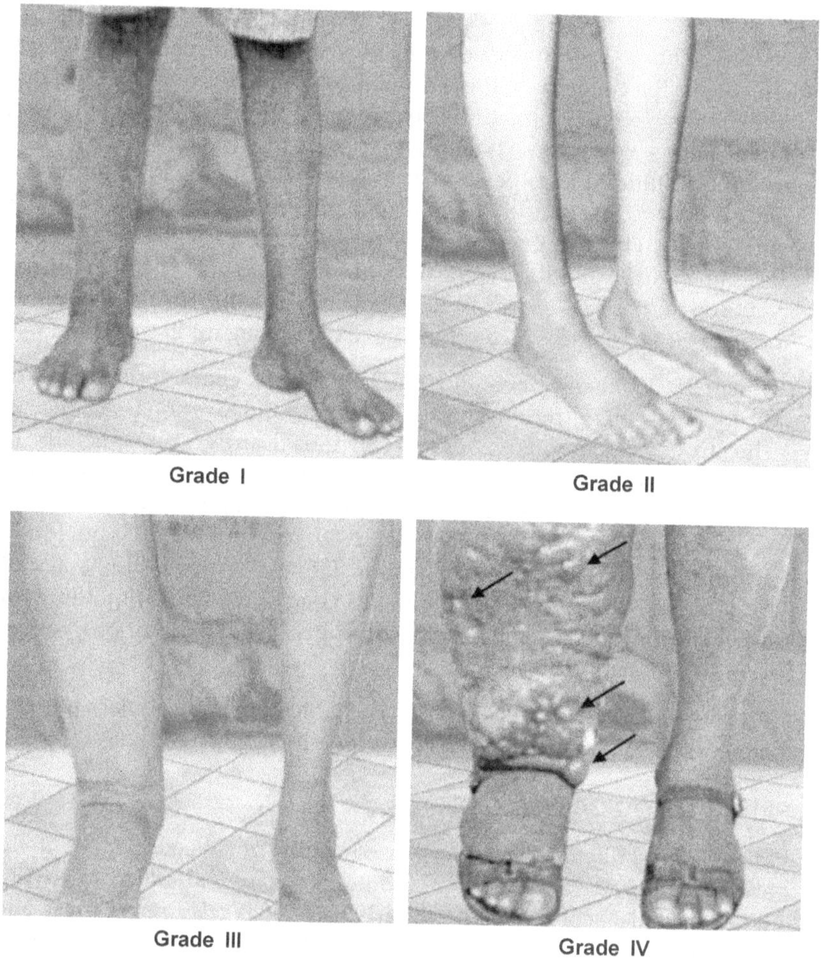

Fig. 28.4: Lymphedema grades of lower extremity

'positive fluctuation' for fluid and a positive transillumination test. Repeated episodes of adenolymphangitis involving the testicular lymphatics (epididymo-orchitis) may precede the development of hydrocele.

Lymphedema of the scrotum and penis: When the superficial lymphatics are affected, the skin of the scrotum and penis becomes edematous. The skin becomes hard, thick and irregular with nodules when it is termed elephantiasis of the scrotum. The lymphedematous penis is sometimes described as ram's horn penis. Lymphedema of the scrotum and penis is not graded like lymphedema of the limbs. However, it is prone to get acute ADL attacks just as lymphedema of the limbs. In females, vulval lymphedema can occur as a result of lymph stasis.

Other Manifestations

Chyluria: This condition is due to the blockage of retroperitoneal lymph nodes below the cysterna chyli as a result of which there is reflux of intestinal lymph into the renal lymphatics. The communication is usually at the level of renal pelvis. When these lymphatics rupture, there is flow of chyle into the urine resulting in the passage of milky white urine with lymph. The condition is painless and intermittent and may be associated with hematuria. Chyluria is generally seen after a fatty meal. There are other causes of chyluria and the diagnosis of filarial etiology is one of exclusion and/or on the basis of demonstration of microfilaria (MF) in blood or urine. About 15% of patients with chyluria have circulating mf in their blood.

Tropical Pulmonary Eosinophilia (TPE): TPE is characterized by dry unproductive cough (more at night), wheezing and exertional dyspnea. It is due to hyper-responsiveness to all filarial antigens, especially to microfilaria derived antigen. High levels of filaria-specific antibodies, especially IgE class, and marked elevation of eosinophils are observed in this condition. The eosinophil count is $>3000/cm^3$. In TPE, mf is not found since the immunological hyper-responsiveness removes this stage of parasite from circulation. X-ray of the chest may show miliary mottlings or increased bronchovascular markings. If untreated, TPE may progress to chronic pulmonary fibrosis.

Filarial granulomata: This condition is characterized by painless lump in the breast, subcutaneous tissue or testicle or lymph node.

PARASITOLOGICAL DIAGNOSIS

Parasitological diagnosis has been based mainly on detection of MF in the peripheral blood samples. With some geographical exceptions (like Andaman and Nicobar islands of India), mf of *Wuchereria bancrofti* and *Brugia malayi* are nocturnally periodic with highest densities of mf in peripheral blood occurring at night and for this reason, blood samples are to be collected during night **(Fig. 28.5)**.

Finger Prick Method

Appropriate staining facility, microscope and a skilled technician are required for this procedure. A thick smear is prepared on a microscope glass slide with 20 µl of finger prick blood. The smear is air dried, dehemoglobinized with ordinary water and dried. The slide is stained with JSB- I stain by keeping it in the stain for two minutes. The excess stain is washed off in running tap water and then air-dried by keeping it in a slanting position before examining under a microscope. The demerit of this method is that it cannot detect low-density parasitemia (practically, 20 µl of blood cannot detect mf if the MF count is less than 100/ml of blood, although the

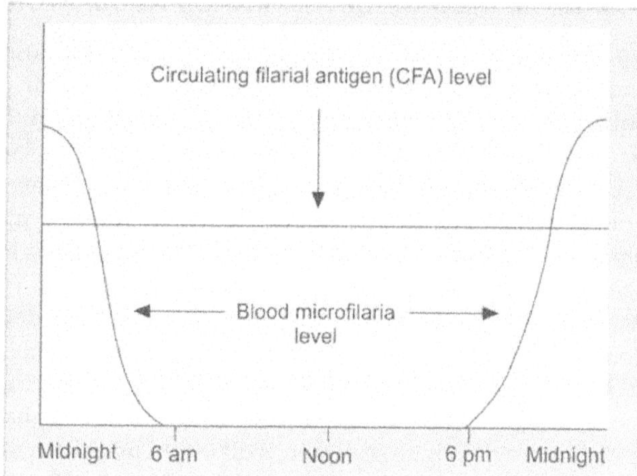

Fig. 28.5: Diurnal variation of blood microfilaria and circulating filaria antigen

theoretical limit is 50/ml). Well-stained specimens are necessary for species identification with characteristic features.

Membrane Filtration Technique

Another method that is commonly used now-a-days in many laboratories is the membrane filtration (MF) technique. One ml of anticoagulated (10% EDTA) venous blood collected at night can be filtered through a polycarbonate membrane (Nucleopore) of 5 µm pore size as described by Dennis and Kean, 1971. Nucleopore membranes are superior to Millipore membranes since the pores are straight through and thus do not clog easily. Use of Millipore requires an elaborate procedure. One ml of anticoagulated (10% EDTA) venous blood collected at night is mixed with 9 ml of Tris EDTA buffer (pH 7.6) in a syringe and is passed through Millipore of 5 µm size. Membrane filter is to be fixed by passing 10 ml of normal saline after which distilled water has to be passed for washing the membrane. The membrane is to be removed from membrane-holder and air-dried and this is followed by staining with JSB-I for 5 minutes as described earlier. Microfilaria can be counted using a microscope. With this technique, even 10 mf/ml can be detected.

Concentration Technique (Knott's)

This technique was originally described by Knott in 1939. One ml of anticoagulated (10% EDTA) venous blood, which was lyzed is fixed by adding 9 ml of 2% formalin in water. After 12 to 24 hours following centrifugation the sediment is stained with methylene blue or Giemsas. However, using formalin increases the amount of sediment. Thus, use of Triton X-100, instead of formalin, reduces the sediment by 84% and saves time for examination.

ULTRASOUND METHOD OF DETECTING OF ADULT WORMS

Visualization of adult worms of *Wuchereria bancrofti in vivo* is possible using ultrasound. Amaral et al., 1994 first demonstrated peculiar pattern of movement (called 'filarial dance sign') of the adult worms in the tubular juxtatesticular dilated lymphatics in male asymptomatic microfilaremic carriers. Later on 'filarial dance sign' of the adult worms was also demonstrated using 7.5 MHz transducer in the testicular lymphatics of asymptomatic microfilaremic carriers. Evidences suggest that ultrasound could even be more sensitive than antigen detection.

Patients can be examined in real-time B mode, using color doppler with a linear, 5.0 or 7.5 MHz transducer. Both sides of the scrotum should be examined serially, first applying the probe to the root of the scrotum and then to the area adjoining the epididymis and testes. The lymphatic vessels and lymph nodes in the inguinal region, axillae and upper arms are also to be examined. Each session of examination can last for about 20 to 30 minutes. Echogenic structures located either in the juxtatesticular lymphatics or lymphatic vessels of spermatic cord can be differentiated from the well recognized turbulence of arterial and venous blood flow. These echogenic structures had a peculiar random but active and localized movement patterns called as filaria dance sign (FDS). These actively motile and linear segments can be observed both in transverse and longitudinal views of the lymphatic vessels. Physical manipulation by pressure will not change the location of FDS suggesting that the structures are localized and stable in these *"filarial nests"*. However, ultrasonography has failed to locate adult worms of *B. malayi in vivo*. This may explain the fact that *B. malayi* infections are not characterized by genital disease whereas hydrocele and epididymo-orchitis are typical of bancroftian disease.

IMMUNODIAGNOSIS

Immunodiagnosis can be based on either detection of specific antibodies or antigens.

Detection of Antibodies

Crude antigens derived from adult worms of *Brugia pahangi* or *Dirofilaria immitis* are used for detection of filarial antibodies. However, these antigens cross react with eight filarial species infecting humans and also with intestinal helminths. Therefore, these tests are of little value in endemic areas; however, these can be used in non-endemic areas for screening purpose.

Detection of *Brugia malayi* specific IgG4 isotype antibodies has been carried out using a recombinant antigen in three endemic countries. This test has shown 95.6 to 100% specificity and 96 to 100% sensitivity, a positive predictive value of 75 to 100% and negative predictive value of 98.9 to 100% when compared with either membrane filtration technique or PCR. This does not cross react with other helminths. This has been marketed as 'Brugia-Rapid dip-stick' method.

Detection of Circulating Filarial Antigen (CFA)

Two tests are available for detection of soluble CFA of *Wuchereria bancrofti*. The first commercially available kit to detect CFA was by 'JCU Tropical Biotechnology'. This test uses a monoclonal antibody, Og4C3 derived by using cattle parasite *Onchocerca gibsoni* antigen in rabbits. CFA is detected using sera samples or from eluted filter paper soaked blood samples by sandwich ELISA. This test gives quantitative results of CFA. The sensitivity of this test varies between 75 to 100% and specificity of 98.4%. It is observed that there is strong correlation between MF density and antigen prevalence. Finger prick day-blood samples soaked in filter paper can be used for detection of CFA by Og4C3 ELISA.

Another species-specific CFA detection test using immunochromatography (ICT) is available and is marketed by "NOW" ICT. The ICT card can be used for serum, plasma and whole blood. A line of monoclonal antibody (gold-labeled) directed against CFA (initially raised against *Dirofilaria immitis*) is present at the top of a nitrocellulose strip that arrests the CFA and forms a visible pink line within five minutes and can be stored as records. The ICT has undergone extensive field tests in different countries. The sensitivity and specificity of ICT varies between 98 to 100% and 93 to 100% respectively when compared to thick blood smear whereas the variation is between 95 to 100% and 94 to 100% respectively when compared to membrane filtration technique. The ICT was developed and manufactured initially by ICT Diagnostics, Brook vale, Australia and later by AMRAD, Frenchs Forest, Australia, and it is currently being produced by Binax, Inc., Portland, and USA and is available as ICT "NOW® ICT Filariasis". Though the formats of the earlier two versions were the same, the latest version is reported to have undergone a significant modification in order to make it more sensitive. However, the basic immunological reagents viz., the *W. bancrofti* specific monoclonal and polyclonal antibodies remain the same in all the versions. The latest version of ICT "NOW® ICT Filariasis" has problem of stability of reaction lines at 10 minute and 24 hours.

MOLECULAR DIAGNOSIS

During the last decade, several polymerase chain reactions have been described which provide species-specific detection of both brugian and bancroftian DNA. Initially only satisfactory use was with night blood. But sensitivity was increased by use of modified primers targeting repetitive DNA sequences such as the SspI repeat or the whole AccI sequence. So detection of *Wuchereria* DNA from diurnally collected blood samples became possible with a sensitivity of 93% (compared to thick films) and 94% (compared to membrane filtration of 1 ml respectively). Both studies report that PCR is able to detect DNA in amicrofilaremic individuals too but a recent study comparing parasitological methods, PCR, Og4C3 ELISA and ultrasound revealed that PCR was neither able to detect DNA in amicrofilaremic but antigen-positive individuals, nor in amicrofilaremic subjects with sonographically visualized adult worms. Sensitivity equaled Nuclepore filtration of 1 ml venous blood. PCR has shown some promise with non-invasive samples, e.g. urine (sensitivity 59.7%) or sputum (sensitivity 94%); however, specificity for sputum remains to be established, since the primers used may cross-react with other nematodes temporarily present in sputum. For brugian filariasis, a more user-friendly procedure using finger prick blood and ELISA detection has been described. This method has 100% sensitivity. Compared to a thick blood smear as the 'gold standard', PCR was positive in 12 times as many cases with specificity of 88%. However, repeated testing giving identical results, indicates that the 'false positives' are probably a consequence of the low sensitivity of the blood smear. The above PCR methods are nonquantitative, primarily because blood samples contain unpredictable amounts of PCR inhibitors.

DIAGNOSIS IN VECTORS

Manual Dissection for L3 Larval Stage of Parasite

Hand caught resting vector *Culex quinquefasciatus* can be dissected and examined under microscope to detect L3 larvae. Detection of infection and infectivity in vectors indicates an area to be endemic with ongoing transmission.

PCR Based Detection of Infection in Vectors

A Hha 1 based polymerase chain reaction (PCR) assay has been developed for the detection of *Brugia malayi*, the causative agent of Brugian lymphatic filariasis. Laboratory studies showed that the new assay was highly sensitive in comparison with the standard dissection and microscopy technique. The assay can detect as little as 4 pg of parasite DNA or a single microfilaria in pools of up to 100 mosquitoes. The optimum pool size for convenience was found to be 50 mosquitoes per pool. A PCR assay based on SspI repeats of *Wuchereria bancrofti* has shown potential in the detection of infection in vectors, *Culex quinquefasciatus*, prevalent in India.

EPIDEMIOLOGY AND PUBLIC HEALTH

Filariasis Problem in India

Globally, about 1,100 million people live in areas endemic for lymphatic filariasis (in 81 countries) and are exposed to the risk of infection; and there are about 120 million cases of filariasis, either having patent microfilaremia or chronic filarial disease. It has been estimated that in India, there are 429 million people exposed to the risk of infection, 31.3 million individuals with patent microfilaremia, and 7.4 million with lymphedema and 12.9 million with hydrocele.

Prevalence, Incidence and Distribution (Fig. 28.6)

Prevalence of infection and disease in human population is measured as proportion infected with detectable microfilaremia (MF rate in %) and proportion with disease (disease rate in %). The endemicity of an area or a given population refers to proportion positive for infected or diseased or both. The prevalence of disease under the national program is recorded as the proportion of population with gross filarial pathology, often detected by health worker questionnaire about lymphedema and hydrocele, rather than by any physical examination. For this reason, the disease prevalence rates reported are expected to be much lower than the disease prevalence (obtained by clinical examination by physician).

Trend of Filariasis Over Course of Time

The estimated population residing in endemic areas and exposed to the risk of infection, persons harboring microfilaria in their blood and persons with disease manifestations in different years (1962–2001) are presented in

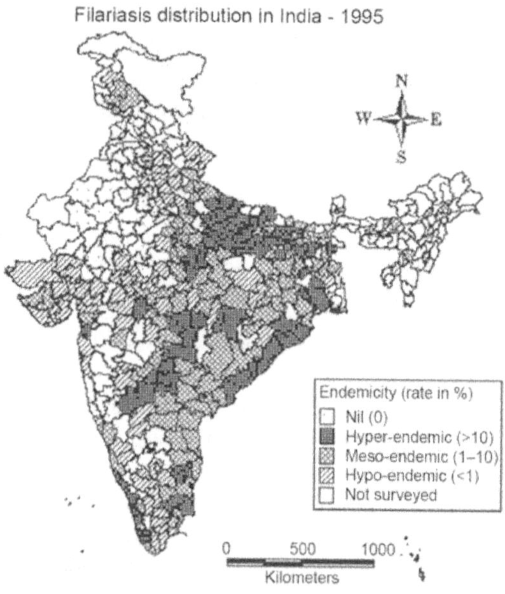

Fig. 28.6: Filariasis endemicity in India

(Table 28.3). The increasing trend observed in these estimates is primarily due to the increasing size of the population and is complemented with rapid urbanization. Apart from this, the changes in land use patterns, the newer water resources development projects, deforestation, rapid urbanization and industrialization and above all the population movement at higher rate could have resulted in the introduction of infection to the newer (non-endemic) areas. A declining trend is observed in high endemic districts in the past four decades and it is partly due to various control measures in vogue in these areas. On the other hand, there is an increase in the number of low and moderate endemic districts and this could reflect the increase in the problem in some rural areas (where there is no control) and that of spread of the disease to newer areas. The microfilaria and disease prevalence in different states of India are shown in **(Tables 28.4 and 28.5)**.

MANAGEMENT

Management of filariasis infection and disease:
- Medical management
- Surgical management
- Physiotherapeutical management.

Medical management
1. Acute filarial disease (limb and genital area)
   - Use of antibiotics recommended in ADL due to secondary bacterial infection and epididymo-orchitis
   - The antibiotic(s) of choice would be penicillin group/macrolides/ gentamycin since the causative organism in most instances is Beta hemolytic streptococci sensitive to the above organisms
   - Supportive treatment including antipyretics, anti-inflammatory drugs, local treatment of entry lesions, rest, limb elevation to be advised

Table 28.3: Filarial infection status at different years in India

	Estimated population at risk of infection (millions)			*Estimated number of cases (millions)*		*Number of cases per 1000 popn. at risk*	
Year	*Rural*	*Urban*	*Total*	*MF*	*Disease*	*MF*	*Disease*
1962	40.16	24.08	64.24	5.0	4.40	7.8	6.8
1970	84.91	51.39	136.30	11.3	8.00	8.3	5.9
1976	174.08	62.05	236.13	18.3	14.40	7.8	6.1
1981	221.92	82.08	304.00	21.7	15.84	7.2	5.2
1985	251.80	90.56	342.36	23.7	17.56	6.9	5.1
1989	275.36	98.94	374.30	25.0	19.00	6.7	5.1
1994	302.87	108.78	411.65	26.9	20.40	6.5	5.0
1995	315.11	113.17	428.28	28.0	21.20	6.5	5.0
2001	NA	NA	472.00	30.9	23.4	6.5	4.8

Table 28.4: *Microfilariae* rates in different states of India

Sl. No.	States/UTs	2004	2005	2006	2007	2008	2009
1.	Andhra Pradesh	1.36	0.74	0.69	0.24	0.38	0.45
2.	Assam	ND	0.04	0.19	1.46	0.88	
3.	Bihar	1.5	2.15	1.38	0.68	NR	
4.	Chhattisgarh	ND	1.96	ND	0.61	0.45	
5.	Goa	0.11	0.04	0.02	0.08	0.01	0.00
6.	Gujarat	0.22	0.84	0.81	0.35	0.83	0.92
7.	Jharkhand	ND	0.84	1.40	1.34	1.10	1.11
8.	Karnataka	1.87	0.84	0.69	1.15	1.07	0.93
9.	Kerala	0.68	0.5	0.67	0.65	0.29	0.39
10.	Madhya Pradesh	0.83	0.4	0.38	0.70	0.36	0.40
11.	Maharashtra	1.13	1.45	1.13	0.83	0.35	0.46
12.	Orissa	2.6	2.37	1.11	0.99	0.74	0.60
13.	Tamil Nadu	0.04	0.38	0.39	0.29	0.15	0.12
14.	Uttar Pradesh	1.77	1.01	0.83	0.32	0.41	
15.	West Bengal	4.74	4.1	2.72	2.83	0.89	0.48
16.	A and N Islands	1.4	0.09	0.15	0.34	0.19	0.46
17.	D and N Haveli	1.96	2.01	2.91	3.47	1.82	1.23
18.	Daman and Diu	0.47	0.14	0.27	0.09	0.13	0.07
19.	Lakshadweep	1.19	0.09	0.07	0.02	0.27	
20.	Pondicherry	0.42	0.5	0.15	0.06	0.03	0.00

- Antifilarial drugs not to be given during an acute attack. However, a standard course of diethylcarbamazine (DEC 6 mg/kg/day in divided doses X 12 days) may be given after the acute phase of filarial adenitis, epididymo-orchitis or acute hydrocele if patients are found to be MF +ve. But these drugs may be started only after the acute symptoms have subsided
- If a patient gets recurrent ADL attacks despite good limb hygiene, prophylactic penicillin either parenteral or oral may be given
  There is no role for diuretics/antihistamines.

2. Tropical pulmonary eosinophilia (TPE)
   - TPE to be diagnosed in a patient presenting with symptoms of dry nocturnal cough and exertional dyspnea and who has an AEC of > 3000 cells or differential eosinophil count of over 25% in the absence of other intestinal helminth infestation.
   - The initial treatment should be with DEC in standard dose of 6 mg/kg/day for three weeks. If there is no response after six weeks of completing the course, a short course of prednisolone (7.5 mg/day for 7 days) to be given. Tapering of the dose is not essential for prednisolone as it is in physiological dose
   - Symptomatic treatment with bronchodilators to be given if required.

Table 28.5: Filarial disease rates in different states of India

	Name	*Surveyed districts*	*Endemic districts*	*Population at risk*	*Diseased*	*Disease prevalence*
1.	Andhra Pradesh	20	20	66459815	2083925	4.57
2.	Arunachal Pradesh	0	0			
3.	Assam	8	8	10343384	62950	0.0
4.	Bihar	25	22	67143944	8086156	1.79
5.	Chhatisgarh	4	4	9774502	149920	
6.	Goa	2	2	1343998	1344	0
7.	Gujarat	19	18	41559362	155663	0.02
8.	Haryana	5	0	3228539	0	
9.	Himachal Pradesh	5	0	s	0	
10.	Jammu and Kashmir	6	0	3384988	0	
11.	Jharkhand	12	12	19632530	490694	
12.	Karnataka	14	12	27046689	169280	7.37
13.	Kerala	10	10	27488468	2500221	1.07
14.	Madhya Pradesh	37	34	45331089	699233	1.26
15.	Maharashtra	13	13	38523081	491486	0.97
16.	Manipur	1	0	393780	0	
17.	Meghalaya	2	0	760099	0	
18.	Mizoram	0	0		0	
19.	Nagaland	1	1	314366	629	
20.	Orissa	12	12	20081380	646598	16.68
21.	Punjab	3	0	752287	0	
22.	Rajasthan	12	0	23493591	0	
23.	Sikkim	0	0		0	
24.	Tamil Nadu	25	23	54151329	1381651	0.05
25.	Tripura	1	0	590655	0	
26.	Uttar Pradesh	47	47	125920212	6093012	6.26
27.	Uttaranchal	6	6	3503788	10537	
28.	West Bengal	14	14	66821769	3721478	11.81
29.	Andaman and Nicobar Islands	2	2	356265	924	0.04
30.	Chandigarh	1	1	900914	0	
31.	Dadra and Nagar Haveli	1	1	220451	220	
32.	Daman and Diu	2	2	158059	225	0.21
33.	Delhi	0	0		0	
34.	Lakshadweep	1	1	60595	0	0
35.	Pondicherry	4	4	942467	1965	0.45
	Grand Total	**315**	**269**	**660682396**	**26748113**	**1.5**

3. Chronic disease–lymphedema without ADL
    - The seven stage classification of WHO does not appear to provide any added benefit in the management. Hence, its utility to a treating physician is negligible
    - Emphasis to be given to limb hygiene and care of entry lesions

- DEC need not be given to chronic lymphedema patients since they would have probably received a course of DEC earlier.
- Among the physical methods, only foot elevation needs to be emphasized
- There is no role for drugs like flurocid injections, coumarins and diuretics. Coumarin should be particularly discouraged because of its hepatotoxicity.

4. Asymptomatic carriers
   - It is essential to treat asymptomatic carriers for the overall benefit to the community.
5. Scrotal swelling
   - Antibiotics and supportive therapy to be given for epididymo-orchitis
   - This was to be followed by a single dose of DEC
   - There was no role for DEC in hydrocele except for mf+ve cases who had to be treated
   - All hydroceles to be referred to surgeons.
6. Chronic disease

The basic components of chronic lymphedema management are hygiene, and elevation. The single most important factor that will help the patients is maintaining good hygiene which includes "limb care" and treating entry lesions.

Limb hygiene ***(Figs 28.7A to C)****:* A very important factor that leads to the progression of the disease is recurrent attacks of ADLA which is mainly due to secondary bacterial infection of the skin and subcutaneous tissue.

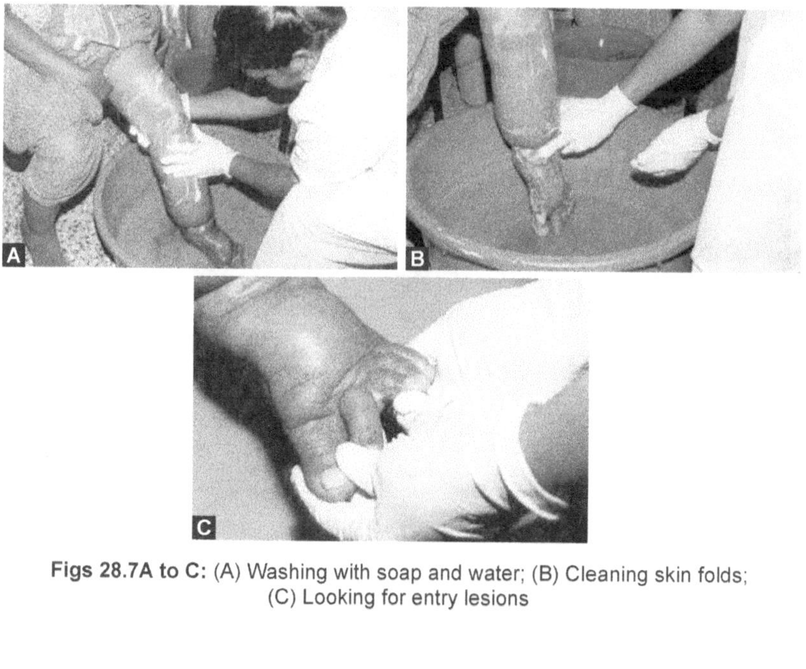

Figs 28.7A to C: (A) Washing with soap and water; (B) Cleaning skin folds; (C) Looking for entry lesions

Therefore it is necessary to prevent acute ADLA attacks to prevent the progression of the disease.

This is done by educating the patient on limb care. Emphasis is laid on limb hygiene and prompt treatment of entry lesions to prevent secondary bacterial infections.

Elevation **(*Figs 28.8A to E*)**: This promotes lymph flow and prevents fluid from accumulating in the leg. Whenever possible the patient should keep his limbs elevated, particularly so in the night while sleeping.

Surgical Management of Lymphedema (Flow chart 28.1)

Principles

- Augment lymphatic drainage
- Reduce the lymphatic load
- Procedure must be physiological.

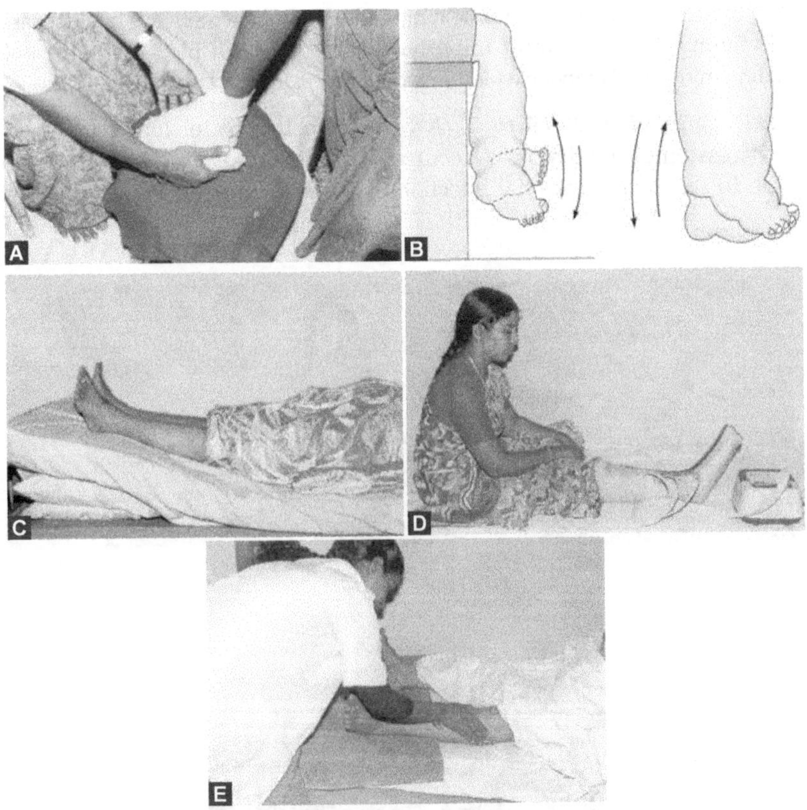

Figs 28.8A to E: (A) Use of pressure bandage; (B) Passive exercise of limb (C) Elevation of limb; (D) Pneumatic compression; (E) Manual massage

Flow chart 28.1: Management of lymphedema cases

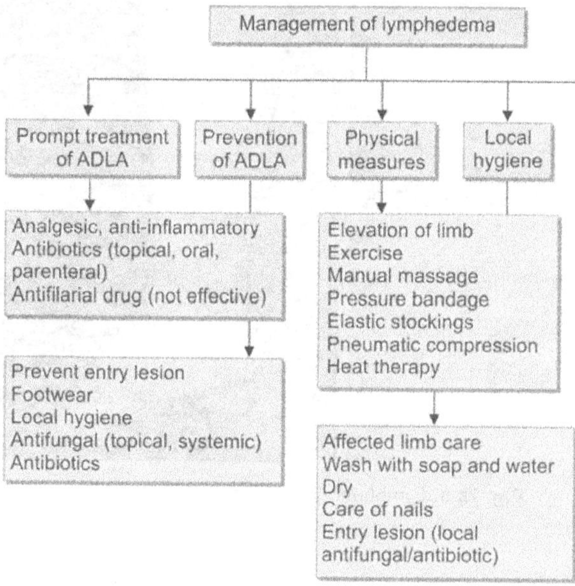

Surgical Methods Available

1. Nodovenous or lymphovenous shunts
2. Microvascular transplantation of free lymph node
3. Free muscle transfer
4. Venous bypass grafts
5. Autogenous transplantation of lymphatic vessels
6. Lympholymphatic anastomoses
7. Laser surgery
8. Lymphosuction

   Nodovenous or lymphovenous shunts **(Figs 28.9 and 28.10A to C)**:

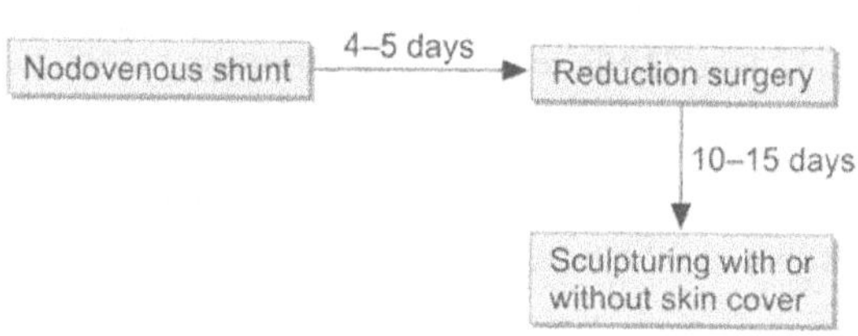

TOWARDS ELIMINATION OF LYMPHATIC FILARIASIS (ELF) IN INDIA

India is committed to elimination of filariasis as it is a signatory to the WHO resolution on the same in 1997. India considered this as a priority in

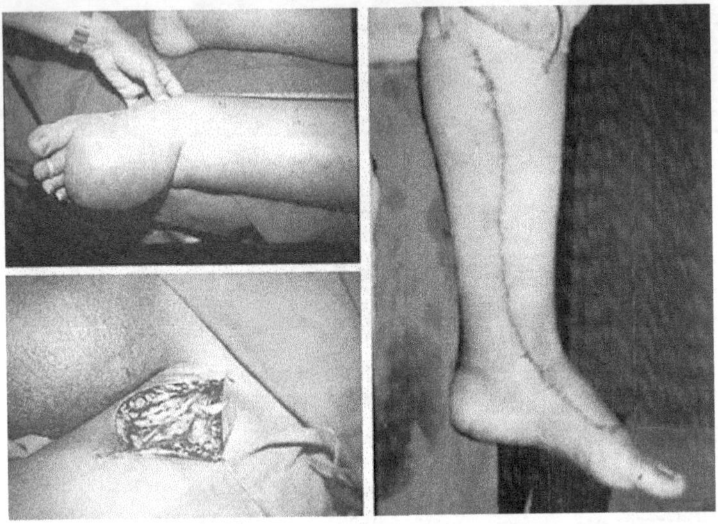

Fig. 28.9: Lymphonodo-venous shunt

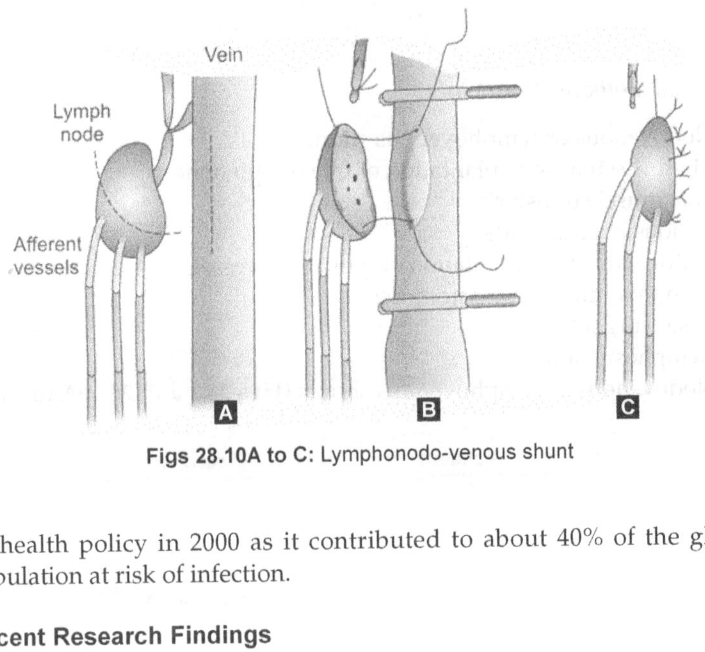

Figs 28.10A to C: Lymphonodo-venous shunt

its health policy in 2000 as it contributed to about 40% of the global population at risk of infection.

Recent Research Findings

- DEC as single annual dose is shown to be safe and effective drug for mass consumption for the control of filariasis. Primarily, DEC is a microfilaricidal drug but is also known to kill up to 50% of the adult.
- Morbidity control-foot hygiene is very effective in the prevention of ADL.

- New simple diagnostic tools (ICT, OG4C3 and DNA probes) are becoming available. These will be of value to evaluate the success of chemotherapy programs directed towards the parasite in humans.

Objectives of ELF

1. To reduce and eliminate transmission of LF by mass drug administration (MDA) of diethylcarbamazine citrate (DEC) or DEC and albendazole.
2. To reduce and prevent morbidity in diseased persons.

The Salient Aspects of ELF Strategy

1. Single day mass therapy with DEC at 6 mg/kg body weight or DEC and albendazole annually.
2. Management of acute and chronic filariasis and self-care methods at doorstep.
3. Antivector measures to continue in all the NFCP towns as complementary to antiparasitic measure and microfilarial carriers (detected in filaria clinics and elsewhere) to receive the standard dose of DEC at 6 mg/kg body weight per day for 12 days.

Transmission Control

Transmission control aims at interruption of transmission by either of the following methods:

- Parasite control
- Vector control
- Reduction in man vector contact.

Parasite control is primarily targeted for reduction in parasite load in human community leading to reduction in transmission, with subsequent reduction in appearance of fresh cases of infection and finally reduction in morbidity in long-term.

Vector control is another means of transmission control, targeting either against immature larval stages using chemical, biological tools or by environmental modification; or adult mosquitoes by using chemical insecticides. In India, larval control is being routinely carried out in the urban areas covered under the program. It has apparently become costly, since it is carried out routinely, without consideration of the vector seasonality and other factors.

Reduction in man vector contact can be in the form of use of mosquito nets or mosquito repellents.

Morbidity Control

Classically, filariasis results in acute adenolymphangitis (ADL), lymphedema leading to gross elephantiasis and hydrocele. Prevention of progression of infection to disease and of episodic ADL attacks will not only be important from the viewpoint of reducing morbidity but also to increase the acceptance of the overall program implementation. Morbidity control/management should therefore form an integral component of the elimination strategy. The frequency of these attacks increases with progression of disease. Due to the functional blockade in lymph flow, secondary bacterial invasion, particularly with Beta hemolytic *streptococci*, results in acute inflammatory ADL. It has also been shown that repeated skin injury, ulceration of the oedematous part, etc. predispose to ADL attacks. The following measures are currently suggested:

- For prevention of ADL attacks foot care/hygiene (and use of antibiotics, particularly long acting penicillin)
- For reduction or arrest of progression of lymphedema, monthly courses of DEC (6 mg/kg/day in 3 divided doses) and community based physiotherapeutic measures including manual massage.

BIBLIOGRAPHY

1. Amaral F, Dreyer G, Figuiredo-Silva J, Cavalcanti A, Samico SC, Santos A, Coutinho A. Live adult worms detected by ultrasonography in human bancroftian filariasis. Am J Trop Med Hyg 1994;50:753-7.
2. Chanteau S, Moulia-Pelat JP, Glaziou P, Nguyen NL, Luquiaud P, Plichart C, Martin PMV, Cartel JL. Og4C3 Circulating Antigen: A marker of infection and Adult worm burden in Wuchereria bancrofti filariasis. Journal of Infectious Disease 1994;170:247-50.
3. Das PK, Ramaiah KD, Vanamail P, Pani SP, Yuvaraj J, Balarajan K. Bundy DAP. Placebo controlled community trial of four cycles of single dose diethyl carbamazine or Ivermectin against Wuchereria bancrofti infection and transmission in India. Trans Roy Soc Trop Med and Hyg (Submitted) 2002.
4. Das PK. Changing environment and its impact on filariasis in India. Proceedings of the National Seminar on Environment and Health. 1998. New Delhi 1998.pp.1-43.
5. Dreyer G, Santos A, Noroes J, Amaral F, Addiss D. Ultrasonographic detection of living adult *Wuchereria bancrofti* using a 3.5 MHz transducer. Am J Trop Med Hyg 1998;59:399-403.
6. Itoh M, Gunawardena NK, Qiu XG, Weerasooriya MV, Kimura E. The use of whole blood absorbed on filter paper to detect *Wuchereria bancrofti* circulating antigen. Transaction of the Royal Society of Tropical Medicine and Hygiene 1998;92:513-5.
7. King CL, Freedman DO. Filarial infection. In: Hunter's Tropical Medicine and emerging infectious diseases. Strickland T, WB Saunders Co (Ed), 8th edn. 1999.pp.750-1.
8. Knott J. A method for making microfilarial surveys on day blood. Trans R Soc Trop Med Hyg 1939;33:191.
9. Lammie PJ, Hightower AW, Eberhard ML. Age specific prevalence of antigenemia in a *Wuchereria bancrofti*-exposed population. American Journal of Tropical Medicine and Hygiene 1994;51:348-55.
10. Lucena WA, Dhalia R, Abath FGC, Nicolas L, Regis LN, Furtado AF. Diagnosis of *Wuchereria bancrofti* infection by the polymerase chain reaction using urine

and day blood samples from amicrofilaraemic patients. Transactions of the Royal Society of Tropical Medicine and Hygiene 1998;92:290-3.

11. McMahon JE, Marshall TFC, Vaughan JP, Abaru DE. Bancroftian filariasis: A comparison of microfilariae counting techniques using counting chamber, standard slide and membrane (nucleopore) filtration. Annals of Tropical Medicine and Parasitology 1979;73:457-64.
12. Melrose WD, Turner PF, Pisters P, Turner B. An improved Knott's concentration test for detection of microfilariae. Transactions of the Royal Society of Tropical Medicine and Hygiene 2000;94:176.
13. Michael E, Bundy DAP, Grenfell BT. Re-assessing the global prevalence and distribution of lymphatic filariasis Parasitology 1996;112:409-28.
14. More SJ, Copeman DB. A highly specific and sensitive monoclonal antibody-based ELISA for the detection of circulating antigen in bancroftian filariasis. Tropical Medicine and Parasitology 1990;41:403-6.
15. Noroes J, Addiss D, Amaral F, Coutinho A, Medeiros Z, Dreyer G. Occurrence of living adult Wuchereria bancrofti in scrotal area of men with microfilaraemia. Transactions of the Royal Society of Tropical Medicine and Hygiene 1996;90:55-6.
16. Ottesen EA, Duke BOL, Karam M, Behbehani K. Strategies and tools for the control/elimination of lymphatic filariasis, WHO Bulletin. 1997;75:49-503.
17. Pani SP, Balakrishnan N, Srividya A, Bundy DAP, Grenfell BT. Clinical epidemiology of bancroftian filariasis: Effect of age and gender. Trans Roy Soc Trop Med and Hyg 1991;85:260-4.
18. Pani SP, Dhanda V. Natural history and dynamics of progression of clinical manifestations of filariasis. In: Proceedings of the CSIR golden jubilee symposium on Tropical disease: Molecular biology and control strategies, CDRI, Lucknow. Kumar S, Sen AK, Dutta GP, Sharma RN (Eds). New Delhi, Publications and Information Directorate CSIR 1994.pp.1-8.
19. Pani SP, Hoti SL, Elango A, Yuvaraj J, Lall R, Ramaiah KD. Evaluation of the ICT whole blood antigen card test to detect infection due to nocturnally periodic Wuchereria bancrofti in South India. Tropical Medicine and International Health 2000;5:359-63.
20. Pani SP, Lall R. Clinical features, pathogenesis and management of lymphatic filariasis, ICMR Bulletin. 1998;28:41–51.
21. Pani SP, Srividya A, Krishnamoorthy K, Das PK, Dhanda V. Rapid Assessment Procedures (RAP) for lymphatic filariasis. National Medical Journal of India 1997a;10:19-22.
22. Pani SP, Srividya A, Rajagopalan PK. Clinical manifestations of bancroftian filariasis in relation to microfilaraemia and diethylcarbamazine therapy. The National Medical Journal of India 1991a;4:9-14.
23. Pani SP, Yuvaraj J, Vijayalakshmi G, Subramanyam Reddy G. Management of lymphatic filariasis – a manual for clinicians. Pondicherry, Vector Control Research Centre 1997.pp.1–22.
24. Pani SP, Yuvaraj J. Epidemiology of filarial lymphedema. Proceeding of 1st nnual Conference of Lymphology Society of India, Thanjavur, India; 1996.pp.11-20.
25. Rahmah N, Ashikin AN, Anuar AK, Ariff RHT, Abdullah B, Cdhan GT, Williams SA. PCR-ELISA for the detection of Brugia malayi infection using finger prick blood. Transactions of the Royal Society of Tropical Medicine and Hygiene. 1998;92:404-6.

26. Rocha A, Addiss D, Ribeiro ME, Noroes J, Baliza M, Medeiros Z, Dreyer G. Evaluation of Og4C3 ELISA in *Wuchereria bancrofti* infection: infected persons with undetectable or ultra-low microfilarial densities. Tropical Medicine and International Health 1996l;1:859-64.
27. Sabesan S, Krishnamoorthy K, Panicker KN, Vanamail P. The dynamics of microfilaraemia and its relation with development of disease in periodic Brugia malayi infection in South India. Epidemiology and Infection 1991;107:453-63.
28. Sabesan S, Palaniyandi M, Das PK, Michael E. Mapping of lymphatic filariasis in India. Annals of Tropical Medicine and Parasitology. 2000.p.94.
29. Subramanyam Reddy G, Das LK, Pani SP. The preferential site of adult Wuchereria bancrofti: An ultrasound study of male asymptomatic microfilaria carrriers in Pondicherry, India. The National Medical Journal of India, vol. 17 2004;(4):195-6.
30. Subramanyan Reddy G, Vengateswarlou N, Das PK, Vanamail P, Vijayan, Sasikala, Pani SP. Single dose diethyl carbamazine (DEC) or Ivermectin in the clearance of Wuchereria bancrofti microfilareamia at Pondicherry, South India. Tropical Medicine and International Health. 2000 (Accepted).
31. Subramanyan Reddy G, Vengateswarlou N. Mass administration of DEC medicated salt for filariasis control in the endemic population of Karaikal, South India; Implementation, Impact Assessment. WHO Bulletin. 1996;74: 85-90.
32. Suresh S, Kumaraswami V, Suresh I, Krishnamurthy R, Ganesan S, Vadivelu V, Arunachalam R, Gopalrajan R. Ultrasonographic diagnosis of sub-clinical filariasis. Journal of Ultrasound Medicine. 1997;16:45-9.
33. Tewari SC, Hiriyan J, Rueben R. Epidemiology of subperiodic *Wuchereria bancrofti* infection in Nicobar islands, India. Trans Roy Soc Trop Med and Hyg 1995;89:163-6.
34. Travancore Cochin state II, Shertallai Taluk. Indian Journal Malariology. 10:203
35. Weil GJ, Lammie PJ, and Weiss N. The ICT Filariasis test: A rapid- format antigen test for diagnosis of bancroftian filariasis. Parasitology Today 1997;13:401-4.
36. WHO. Lymphatic filariasis: the disease and its control. Fifth report of the WHO expert committee on filariasis. WHO Technical Report Series 1992;821: 1-67.
37. WHO. The application of modelling to control strategies in lymphatic filariasis: report of a consultative meeting. TDR/AFR/FIL97. 1997a;1:1-23.
38. WHO. The state of World health, The world health report 1995: Bridging the gap, Report of the Director General; 1995.pp.1-48.

29 Chapter
Cryptosporidiosis and Cyclosporiasis

JK Dutta

CRYPTOSPORIDIOSIS

Cryptosporidium was first described in 1907, but first case of human infection was recorded in 1976. It is a gastrointestinal coccidian protozoa. It is widely distributed globally and has 10 species. *C parvum* is responsible for most of human infections. *C.felis* infects mostly children. *C.parvum* is known to be infectious in more than 150 mammals including man.

Mode of Infection

The infection spreads by feco-oral route through oocyst-contaminated water, food or by personal contact with man infected with *C. parvum.* Transmission through infected, uncooked vegetables, cider, apple juice, chicken salad and shell fish is possible. Infection occurs during late summer among all age groups but more often in persons below 20 years of age. The infection is of special concern in immune-suppressed states like HIV infection and malignancy and in elderly persons in whom treatment may be difficult. Transplant recipients are also vulnerable to the infection.

Clinical Features

The incubation period varies from 2 to 14 days with a median period of 7 days. The main symptom is diarrhea. Explosive diarrhea with dehydration may occur in AIDS patients. Other symptoms which accompany diarrhea include abdominal cramp, vomiting, nausea, loss of appetite, aching in muscle and joint pain. In some patients, arthritis, conjunctivitis and erythema of oral mucosa may be evident. Extra-intestinal infection can occur which may result in pancreatitis, hepatitis, cholangitis and pulmonary infection. Cryptosporidium oocysts may be excreted. In some persons, excretion may be intermittent. So, at least three stool samples must be examined at interval of few days.

Diagnosis

The current methods of diagnosis include identification of the oocysts in stool specimen. Three staining methods are available which include auramine staining, modified Ziehl-Nielsen staining and immunofluorescence by using monoclonal antibody to oocysts.

Treatment

The disease is self-limited in immuno-competent persons for whom no chemotherapy is needed. During the attack of diarrhea, fluid and electrolyte balance should be maintained by oral rehydration solution or by use of intravenous saline. No drug is highly effective to control the infection. Nitazoxanide is effective against C. *Parvum* infection. Adult dose is 500 mg to 1 g orally twice daily for 3 days in non-immunocompromised individuals. Children under 4 years should receive 100 mg twice daily for 3 days orally. In advanced AIDS, same dose is given for 2 to 8 weeks. Paromomycin has modest effect only. Dosage is 25 to 35 mg/kg orally for 14 days.

Prevention

Boiled water should be used for drinking purpose. Swimming in public swimming pools should be avoided. The oocysts are resistant to many disinfectants but boiling is an effective method of inactivation. Freezing and drying also inactivate the pathogens.

CYCLOSPORIASIS

In mid 1980s a new pathogen was identified in the stool of some patients suffering from persistent diarrhea. The organism was named as cyclospora cayetanensis. It is a member of the *coccidian genus cyclospora*. It is an emerging parasitic pathogen which is both food and water borne. Cyclospora diarrhea is now widespread in America, Africa, Bangladesh, Australia, South-East Asia, England and Eastern Europe among AIDS patients. The first water borne outbreak was reported in 1995 in USA.

Clinical Features

Diarrhea is persistent and may continue for one to eight weeks along with abdominal pain, nausea, vomiting, anorexia and flatulence. Prolonged diarrhea may lead to profound loss of weight. Episodes of diarrhea may alternate with constipation. There may be cycles of remission and relapse.

Diagnosis

The oocysts can be detected in stool by light microscopy. The parasite can be identified in small-intestinal biopsy material by transmission light microscopy.

Treatment

Trimethoprim-sulfamethoxazole (TMP/SMX) 160 to 800 mg twice daily orally for seven days is the standard treatment. Ciprofloxacin can be used as an alternative drug for persons sensitive to TMP-SMX.

Prevention

Boiled water should always be used for drinking purpose. This advice should be strictly followed by the travelers. TMP-SMX can be used for chemoprophylaxis for immunocompromised patients.

BIBLIOGRAPHY

1. Connolly GM, Dryden MS, Shanson DC, Gazzard BG. Cryptosporidial diarrhoea in AIDS and its treatment. Gut 1988;29:593-7.
2. Rabold JG, Hoge CW, Shilm DR, Kepford C, Rajah R, Echeverria P. Cyclospora outbreak associated with chlorinated drinking water. Lancet 1994;344:1360-1.
3. Soave R, Herewaldt BL, Relman DA. Cyclospora. Infectious Diseases Clinics of North America 1998;12:1-12.
4. Taylor AP, Davis LJ, Soave R. Cyclospora. Current Clinical Topics in infectious Diseases 1997;17:256-68.
5. Tzipori S. Cryptosporidiosis in perspective. Adv Parasitol 1998;27:63-129.

30 Chapter

West Nile Virus, Marburg Virus, Legionellosis

JK Dutta

WEST NILE VIRUS

In August 1999 a physician from Queens, a borough of New York city reported two cases of unusual encephalitis. Soon more cases were detected. At the same time public health officials noted an increase in fatality among New York City birds, particularly the crows. On testing of autopsy specimen of birds, presence of west Nile virus sequence was found by genomic analysis.

VIRUS

West Nile virus is an arbovirus of the family flaviviridae. The virus was first isolated from a woman in the West Nile Province of Uganda in 1937.

The principal vectors are mosquitoes that feed on birds such as *culex pipiens, Aedes* and *Anopheles*. Occasionally ticks also act as vectors. Birds are the principal hosts. A wide variety of animals may be infected by the virus such as raccoons, cats, squirrel, bat and rabbits.

CLINICAL FEATURES

In most of the infected people there is no illness. In some cases fever (flu like illness), malaise, myalgia, sore throat and lymphadenopathy (on the trunk, extremities and head) appear. Signs of aseptic meningitis, encephalitis with confusion, convulsion and coma are observed. Hepatosplenomegaly, pancreatitis, myocarditis are the other manifestations. No specific treatment is available. Mosquito control program is an effective method of prevention.

MARBURG VIRUS

In 1967 a laboratory worker in Marburg, Germany became ill and was hospitalized. He was processing kidney tissues from imported African green monkeys for cell culture and vaccine production. Other cases were also reported same time from Frankfurt (Germany) and Belgrade. It was revealed that monkeys were the source. These monkeys had been imported in one batch from Uganda. A full, investigation ultimately led to the recognition of a new family of virus (Filoviridae) of which Marburg was first recognized. It is an RNA virus and is similar to Ebola virus both genetically and morphologically. It spreads by direct contact with body secretion, excreta, or contaminated equipment. The virus is found in seminal fluid and has been transmitted by sexual contact. Incubation period is 5 to 10 days which is followed by sudden onset of fever, chill, headache and myalgia. Around the fifth day of onset, a maculopapular rash appears on the trunk. Other symptoms include nausea, vomiting, jaundice, pancreatitis, abdominal pain, liver failure, massive hemorrhage and multiorgan failure. Recovery is slow which may be followed by sequelae like orchitis, hepatitis or transverse myelitis. Case fatality rate is 23 to 25%.

Treatment

There is no specific treatment. Supportive measures include fluid and electrolyte replacement as required. Transfusion of blood components may be necessary. Proper barrier-nursing is essential.

LEGIONELLOSIS

In July 1976 an outbreak of a severe form of pneumonia occurred in USA. A previously unknown pathogen was detected in autopsy lung specimen at the center for Disease Control and Prevention. The new pathogen was named as *Legionella pneumophila* and the illness caused by it was termed *Legionnare's* disease.

Etiology

The organism *L. pneumophila* is a gram-negative, aerobic, uncapsulated bacillus. Already 42 species and 64 serotypes of this pathogen have been identified. *L. pneumophila* causes more than 90% of cases of Legionnaire's disease in USA and Europe. *L. longbeachae, L. micdadei, L. dumoffii* and *L. osemanii* are the other known species.

Clinical Features

The incubation period is 2 to 10 days. Two distinct clinical syndromes are caused by the organism—Legionnaire's disease and Pontiac fever.

In the former there is fever, watery diarrhea, unproductive cough and a severe form of pneumonia. The susceptibility is high among immunocompromised persons, elderly people, smokers and persons under immunosuppressive drug therapy.

Pontiac fever has an incubation period of 24 to 48 hours. The first outbreak of Pontiac fever was reported in 1978 in Pontiac, Michigan, USA. It is a comparatively mild illness which is self-limited and nonfatal. There is flu-like illness with malaise, fever, headache and myalgia. Usually there is no evidence of pneumonia.

Diagnosis

Several methods can be used for diagnosis of Legionnaire's disease. Culture of the organism from respiratory secretions is a very suitable method. The culture technique can detect all species of *Legionella*. However, special media are required for culture. Urinary antigen testing is another suitable method. This technique can detect *L. pneumophila* serogroup in over 70% cases. Direct fluorescent antibody test (DFA) is also available for diagnosis. Serological tests are useful for epidemiological studies only. A fourfold rise in antibody titre of acute and subsequent samples is highly suggestive of infection. A single titre of 1:128 provides presumptive evidence of infection.

TREATMENT

Currently available antibiotics like azithromycin, clarithromycin and other macrolides are effective. They can achieve high intracellular concentration. Ciprofloxacin, trovofloxacin and levofloxacin are also useful as they can achieve high pulmonary concentration.

BIBLIOGRAPHY

1. After Marburg Ebola. Lancet 1977;1:581-2.
2. American society of Heating and Air-conditioning Engineers. (ASHRAE) guidelines. 12-2000. Minimizing the risk of Legionellosis associated with building water system (2000), Atlanta, GA. Center for Disease Control and Prevention. Summary of notifiable diseases, United States 1998. MMWR 1999;47(53):1-93.
3. Balter M. On the trail of Ebola and Marburg viruses Science. 2000;290:293-95.
4. Center for disease control and prevention. Fact sheet. Marburg haemorrhagic fever 1999 (on line). Available (tip) www.edc.1 gov ncidod/evrd/sple/mnpages/disinfo/htm.
5. Center for Disease control and Prevention. Outbreak of west Nile-like virus encephalitis-New York 1999. MMWR 1999;48:845-9.
6. Craven RB, Rochrig JT. West Nile virus. J Am Med Assoc 2001;286:651-3.
7. Smith DH, Johnson BK, Isagson, et al. Marburg- virus disease in Kenya. Lancet 1982;1:816-20.
8. World Health Organization. Legionnaire's disease in Europe 1009. Weekly epidemiological record. 1998;73:257-62.
9. World Health Organization. Outbreak news. Legionellosis. Australia (update). Weekly Epidemiological Record. 2000;75:173.

31 Chapter

Lyme Disease and Babesiosis

JK Dutta

LYME DISEASE

In November 1975, a mother in old Lyme, Connecticut, USA reported a cluster of 12 cases with symptoms resembling juvenile rheumatoid arthritis. Investigations indicated that it was a new and previously unrecognized clinical illness and named it as Lyme disease.

Etiology

Lyme disease is caused by a gram-negative spirochete *Borrelia burgdorferi* that is transmitted to human by the tick lxodes scapularis. Mice and deer make up the major animal reservoir of *Borrelia burgdorferi*. The disease is notifiable in USA since 1991. The disease is now prevalent in several countries in Europe, Asia, and Australia besides USA. In USA high incidence is reported from Missouri, North Carolina, Vermont, New Hampshire, Oklahoma, New York, Pennsylvania, Maryland, New Jersey and few other areas.

Clinical Features

Initially a macule or papule appears at the site of tick bite which gradually expands over days or week to form a large round lesion with partial central clearing. The first stage of localized erythema migrans is followed by stage 2 when there is evidence of disseminated infection in other systems. There may be fever, malaise, headache, myalgia, anorexia and intermittent arthralgia. The symptoms may automatically subside for sometime even without any treatment.

In the next stage there are full-fledged manifestations of arthritis and cardiac or neurological symptoms. Arthritis is the most important manifestation which is generally asymmetric and oligoarticular. The knee is mostly involved in about 6 months of initial infection. If left untreated neurological manifestations develop which include headache, photophobia, peripheral neuropathy, facial nerve palsy or encephalopathy. Late neurological syndromes occurring several years after infection may be evident. Chronic lyme disease or post-lyme syndrome has been described but this concept is controversial. Diagnosis can be confirmed by serological tests or by isolation of the organism.

Treatment

Doxycycline 100 mg twice daily or amoxicillin 500 mg three times a day can be used for 14 to 21 days. A vaccine is available for 15 to 70 year age group of persons who live in endemic areas.

BABESIOSIS

Babesiosis is a zoonotic disease caused by protozoal parasites of the genus, Babesia. Because of pear-like appearance, they are also known as piroplasms. More than 100 species are known. *Babesia microti* is the most common infectious agent in man. A new strain Babesia WA-1 has also infected human beings in West Coast of USA. MO-I strain, *Babesia bovis* and *B. divergens* also cause human infection in different countries, particularly in Europe. In USA, Babesiosis is recorded often in Massachusetts, Connecticut, New York and Wisconsin areas.

The usual vector is tick, lxodes scapularis. In Europe lxodes ricinus is the common vector. White-footed mice are the common reservoirs. Mice, rats, bats, certain birds and lizards are frequent hosts.

Clinical Features

Incubation period is usually one to several weeks. Asplenic or immuno-compromised persons are the frequent victims. The disease may also develop after blood transfusion. In such cases the incubation period is shorter. *Babesia* invades the erythrocytes which results in hemolytic anemia. The patient usually develops fever, chill, malaise, sweating, headache and myalgia. Some patients also suffer from nausea, vomiting, abdominal pain, arthralgia, and depression. Some patients pass dark urine. Mild hepatosplenomegaly may be evident. Diagnosis can be confirmed by blood smear examination, serology and PCR. The parasite in the blood smear may be confused with *Plasmodium falciparum*.

Complications

Myocardial infarction, pulmonary edema, respiratory distress syndrome and disseminated intravascular coagulation are the notable complications. Renal failure may be terminal event in some patients which is followed by death.

Treatment

Combination therapy with atovaquone and azithromyin is an effective method of treatment and has few adverse reactions. Exchange transfusion is also a recommended method of treatment. Concurrent infection with Lyme disease is common for which adequate investigations should be carried out. Tick-bite should be avoided which will help to prevent infection.

BIBLIOGRAPHY

1. Center for Disease Control and Prevention. Lyme Disease- United States 1999. MMWR. 2001;50:181-5.
2. Gelfand JA, Challahan MV. Babesiosis. Current Clinical Topics in Infectious Diseases. 1998;18:201-16.
3. Krause PJ, Lepore J, Sikand VK, et al. Atovaquone and azithromycin for the treatment of Babesiosis. New England J Med 2000;343:1454-8.

32 Chapter Creutzfeldt-Jakob Disease

JK Dutta

In 1994, a 19-year-old man in England suffered from depression, hallucination, loss of coordination and gradually failed to walk, talk. He died in May 1995. He became the first victim of "mad-cow" disease (Bovine spongiform encephalopathy).

In March 1996, it was announced by British Government that 10 persons were suffering from Creutzfeldt-Jakob disease (CJD). A link was established between eating beef from cows suffering from bovine spongiform encephalopathy (BSE) and developing the disease. Altered prions were believed to be responsible as the cause.

The original illness described by HG Creutzfeldt and AM Jakob had only some phenotypical features common to what is now conventionally being accepted as CJD. In this disease there are spongiform changes with deposition of amyloid prion protein in the gray matter of the brain. A similar disease is also observed in sheep and goat which is known as "Scrapie". The diseased animals usually scrape or rub and hence the name (scrapie).

ETIOLOGY

Though several authorities believe that the etiological agent is like a virus, most authors are of opinion that the causative agent is a 'prion' protein. Prion protein (PrP) is devoid of nucleic acid and is resistant to enzyme, unlike normal protein. Prion proteins are described as components of the neuronal cell membrane. The usual prion protein is known as Pr Pc (C for cellular). The abnormal form or isoform is known as Pr Psc (sc for scrapie) or Prp Res (Resistant) or P PcJD (cJD for Cr Jakob disease). Prion Protein is genetically coded by prion protein gene (PRNP).

Bovine spongiform encephalopathy (BSE) was first identified in cattle in UK in 1986. It resembled 'scrapie', a transmissible spongiform encephalopathy which affected sheep in England about 2000 years ago.

Classification

CJD occurs in 4 forms—sporadic, familial, iatrogenic and new variant (vCJD). The classical form of CJD was first described in 1920 by two German neurologists.

Sporadic CJD (sCJD)

Approximately 85 to 90% cases of CJD are sporadic in nature. The mean age of onset is 55 to 65 years. Man to man transmission does not occur. In this form of the disease there is neuronal cell death with spongifrom changes, vacuolation and reactive astrocytosis. Amyloid plaques may be seen in some cases.

The onset may be sudden or may be insidious over weeks. Dementia, behavioral changes, myoclonus, cerebellar ataxia, delusion and speech abnormalities develop as signs and symptoms of the disease. It is postulated that the clinical picture depends ultimately on the prion strain or varying prion gene mutation. Hence there may be varied clinical manifestations. There is no specific treatment and no cure.

Iatrogenic CJD

About 5% of all cases of CJD develop this form of the disease. It has been documented to follow dura mater transplantation in neurosurgery. Nearly 80 cases have been recorded. An outbreak of epidemic proportion was observed in Japan among recipients of dural transplant. By now more than 70 cases have been associated with transplantation of dura mater. The disease has developed after use of contaminated surgical instruments and stereotactic depth electroencephalographic electrodes. Some persons developed the disease after use of human pituitary gonadotrophin and intramuscular injection of growth hormone. Nearly 100 cases have been reported who developed CJD due to transmission via pituitary hormone.

Familial CJD

In this form of disease the onset is earlier and the duration is longer. There are at least 11 known mutations in the PRNP gene. It is inherited as autosomal dominant trait and accounts for 5 to 10% of cases of CJD. Gerstmann-Straussier-Scheinker syndrome (GSS) and fatal familial insomnia (FFI) are considered to be variants of this form of disease.

Variant Creutzfeldt-Jakob Disease (vCJD)

In early 1996 a distinct clinical syndrome was identified in ten persons which was a previously unrecognized variant of CJD. This was named variant CJD (vCJD).

The first case was reported in UK. Till June 2004, 154 cases have been reported out of which majority were from UK. Clinical manifestations usually are observed in limbs but face and other parts may be involved. The average age for most cases is 29 years and the duration of illness is longer (average 14 months).

Psychiatric disturbances like depression, schizophrenia and other psychoses are prominent. Abnormal prion proteins have been identified in tonsils of vCJD patients. Criteria for diagnosis of vCJD are as follows.

1. Patient must have a psychiatric illness for at least six months.
2. Patient must have four of the following five...
   a. Ataxia
   b. Depression
   c. Dementia
   d. Persistent painful sensation
   e. A movement disorder (myoclonus, chorea or dystonia).

Extensive 'florid' amyloid plaques are seen in brain with spongiform changes in surrounding areas. World Health Organization has released on May 17, 2001 a revised case definition for vCJD. Progressive neuropsychiatric disorder and neuropathological confirmation are considered to be features of "Definite" vCJD. In fact pathological examination of brain or tonsils can confirm the diagnosis. In most cases there is an abnormal signal on MRI in the FLAIR and diffusion weighted images: a bright one on the thalamus and often less bright ones on the neurocortex and basal ganglia.

CJD cases in India

The number of cases recognized in India was 63 during the period 1980-2000 which were distributed throughout the country. Some of them were vegetarians in whom the mode of infection remained obscure. Highest number of cases was observed in the age group 56 to 65 years. Only one patient was a child of 2 years old. In most of the patients the duration of illness was between three and six months. In 98.7% cases dementia was observed. Myoclonus was the next prominent manifestation (91.0%). Characteristic periodic complexes in EEG were noted in 84.9% patients. In other patients only diffuse slowing was evident in EEG.

Diagnosis

The diagnosis can be confirmed only after pathological examination of brain and tonsils. Amyloid plaques are seen especially more prominently in cases of vCJD. Western blot analysis using cerebral cortex can demonstrate accumulation of proteinase- resistant prion protein (PRNP). PRNP can be demonstrated by PCR technique.

Brain imaging is also a promising diagnostic tool. Thalamus and basal ganglia hyperintensity is the most common abnormality. Familial CJD can be confirmed by prion protein gene analysis on peripheral leucocyte DNA. EEG is a very useful and noninvasive diagnostic method for diagnosis of CJD. The most characteristic features include appearance of 0.5-2 HZ generalized biphasic or triphasic periodic complexes of spikes or sharp waves of 100 to 600 milliseconds duration which are observed in 60-80% patients.

In CSF, proteins are slightly elevated in one-third of patients of CJD. PrP is not consistently detected but other protein markers like 14-3-3 proteins, S-100 proteins, neuron-specific enolase (NSE) and Tau proteins can be identified. Out of these, 14-3-3 has shown the most consistent results in sCJD patients.

Treatment

No effective treatment is available for treatment of CJD in man. However Amphotericin B has been found to reduce PrP concentration in animals. In mice, keratinase has been found effective. In a very recent trial, Flupirtine has shown favorable effect. Genetherapy to prevent production of prion protein when available will be very helpful for treatment. The animals that have developed transmissible spongiform encephalopathy (TSE) should be excluded from human or animal food chain.

Prevention

In UK blood from donors who are residents of affected country is filtered to eliminate the leukocytes which have been implicated as carrier of infection. Appropriate disinfection and sterilization of instruments used during neurosurgical procedures is essential. Guidelines for transfusion of blood and blood products have been revised and enforced in many countries including USA. WHO has also issued guidelines for protection of health care workers and morticians from inadvertent infection.

Adequate infection control in hospitals is mandatory as breaches in infection control have resulted in transmission of some cases. In Great Britain disposable instruments are used for all adenotonsillectomy procedures.

Import of cattle and cattle products should be banned from BSE infected countries. Donors of cornea, liver, dura mater and pituitary extracts should be carefully screened to ascertain absolute freedom from prion protein.

Effective surveillance is necessary to prevent the menace of CJD, vCJD and BSE. In India National Institute of Communicable Disease (NICD) New Delhi, NIMHANS, Bangalore and Neurology Departments of various medical colleges and other leading institutions have been included in the surveillance network.

BIBLIOGRAPHY

1. Alter M. How is Creutzfeldt-Jakob disease acquired? Neuroepidemiology 2000;19:55-61.
2. Amor S, Mehta S. Prions, Viruses and antiviral drugs. Lancet. 1993;342:545.
3. Anonymous Rapidly Progressive dementia in a patient who received cadaveric dura mater graft. MMWR 1987;36:49-50.
4. Batesman D, Hilton D, Love S, et al. Sporadic Creutzfeldt-Jakob disease in an 18-year-old in UK. Lancet. 1995;346:1155-6.
5. Brown P. Bovine spongiform encephalopathy and variant Creutzfeldt-Jakob disease. Br Med J 2001;322:841-4.
6. Creutzfeldt HG. Uber eine eigernatige herdformige ErknanKung des Zentrel inervensystems. Z Gesamte Neurol Psychiatr 1920;57-1.
7. Ferguson-Smith MA. BSE and variant CJD. Assumption that BSE originated from "Scrapie" in sheep led to misjudgement. Br Med J 2001;322:1544-5.
8. Gajdusek DC, Gilebs CJ Jr. Transmission of two subacute spongiform encephalopathies of man (Kuru and Creutzfeldt-Jakob Disease) to New World Monkeys. Nature. 1971;230:588-91.
9. Garil McBride. Contaminated cadaveric dura grafts continue to cause iatrogenic CJD. Neurology Today 2004;3:45.
10. Creutzfeldt-Jakob disease associated with cadaveric duramater grafts-Japan, January 1979-May 1996. MMWR 1997;46:1066-9.
11. Pruisner SB. Novel Proteinaceous infectious particles cause Scrapie. Science 1982;216:136-44.
12. World Health Organization. New case definition for variant CJD. Communicable Diseases Surveillance and Response (CSR). http:11/ www.who.int/emc/diseases/bse/index-html.
13. World Heath Organization. Variant Creutzfeldt-Jakob disease (vCJD). Fact sheet No. 180, 2001.

33 Chapter HIV/TB Coinfection

T Talukdar

INTRODUCTION

Tuberculosis (TB) is the most common opportunistic infection in HIV-infected patients as well as is the leading cause of death. HIV-infected persons are at markedly increased risk for primary or reactivation tuberculosis and for second episodes of tuberculosis from exogenous reinfection. Similarly HIV also has a substantial effect on the incidence, clinical manifestations, treatment and outcome of TB. In fact the escalating tuberculosis case rates seen worldwide over the past two decades are largely attributable to HIV. Coinfection with these pathogens has been devastating in the developing world, especially Sub-Saharan Africa where the burden of disease is high. Without proper treatment, 90% of people living with HIV die within months of contracting TB in this region.

Since a third of the world's population is infected with *Mycobacterium tuberculosis* and more than a half of which lives in countries ravaged by HIV / AIDS, both are crippling the already stretched health care facilities in certain underprivileged countries. Thus together they are better known as the "Deadly Duo or the Dual Epidemic". The World Health Organization (WHO) reports 9.2 million new cases of TB in 2006 of whom 7.7% were HIV-infected. Newer estimates suggest that there were 1.4 million HIV positive TB patients globally in 2008 and over 500,000 people died of HIV-associated TB in 2008. Around 78% of these patients live in Sub-Saharan Africa.

In India, there were 2.5 million people living with HIV and AIDS (PLWHA) at the end of 2007 while the incidence of TB was approximately 1.8 million cases per year. A fifth of all new TB cases worldwide occur here and two in every five Indians have latent TB infection. The HIV seroprevalance in patient of tuberculosis in India varies widely from region to region and is around 5%. This situation differs from that in sub-Saharan Africa, where the incidence of tuberculosis in HIV patients in many countries is much higher than in India and as many as 80% of patients with tuberculosis are coinfected with HIV. In Africa, HIV has reversed the gains in tuberculosis control which started occurring two decades ago.

Increasing prevalence of HIV not only makes diagnosing TB more difficult but also alters the cure rates and increases default and relapse rates. Extrapulmonary, disseminated and sputum smear negative tuberculosis, which are more difficult to diagnose are common in patients with advanced immunosuppression. Treatment of HIV-TB coinfection is associated with the challenges of high pill burden, overlapping drug toxicities, risk of immune reconstitution inflammatory syndrome (IRIS) and maintaining sustained patient compliance.

Thus WHO has brought in the concept of The Three 'I's for TB/HIV (Isoniazid preventive therapy, intensified case finding for TB, and infection control) which will reduce the burden of TB among people living with HIV and therefore must be urgently implemented by all HIV services. WHO in association with the Stop TB Partnership has formed the TB/HIV Working Group which recommends:

- Offer HIV testing and counseling to all TB patients
- Screen all people living with HIV for TB disease
- Provide TB treatment or preventive therapy to all coinfected people
- Provide co-trimoxazole and antiretroviral treatment to all TB patients with HIV
- Ensure TB infection control in all health care facilities and high HIV prevalence settings.

HOW HIV AND TB AFFECTS EACH OTHER

HIV is known to increase the likelihood of developing *Mycobacterium tuberculosis* infection in those uninfected, it is also the most important known risk factor that promotes progression to active TB in people with *Mycobacterium tuberculosis* infection. This risk of progression to active TB disease is 10% annually in comparison to those not infected with HIV, who have a life time risk of only 10%. This progression is also far more rapid, with up to 40% of those developing active TB disease in HIV infected do so within weeks of getting infected. HIV also significantly increases the morbidity and mortality due to active TB disease as compared to those without HIV infection. HIV also increases the incidence of adverse drug reaction and emergence of drug resistance in those receiving antitubercular therapy.

The Th1 class of CD4 T helper cells plays the major role in body's immune response to tuberculosis by producing Interferon gamma. Interferon gamma "activates" the macrophages resulting in phagocytosis of tubercle bacilli and subsequent granuloma formation. HIV infection results in progressive depletion and dysfunction of CD4 lymphocytes. It also results in impaired macrophage function with decreased chemotaxis and defective granuloma formation. Thus HIV infection results in impaired phagocytosis and intracellular killing of the bacilli.

HIV coinfection also makes diagnosing TB more challenging due to frequently negative sputum smears, atypical radiographic presentation, higher prevalence of extrapulmonary TB and other opportunistic pulmonary infections with similar presentations.

Active TB accelerates the course of HIV infection. Immune activation by TB results in enhanced local and systemic HIV replication. *Mycobacterium tuberculosis* increases HIV replication by inducing macrophages to produce tumor necrosis factor alpha, interleukin-1, and interleukin-6. In pulmonary tuberculosis it has been found that the concentrations of HIV RNA are highest in areas of lung with tuberculous involvement.

TB is associated with a 5- to 160-fold increase in HIV viral replication, which decreases after successful TB treatment. This increased replication is mediated through activation of the transcription factors NF-KB and nuclear factor IL-6 due to tubercular infection.

As the CD4 counts fall progressively the risk for opportunistic infections and death becomes higher in HIV/TB coinfected persons than in HIV-infected persons without TB. Thus TB shortens the survival of patients afflicted with HIV infection, by accelerating the progression of HIV and is the cause of death in at least one-third of people with AIDS worldwide. The risk of death in HIV-infected patients with tuberculosis was reported to be twice of that in HIV-infected patients without tuberculosis, independent of the CD4 cell count. This higher mortality is due to the progression of AIDS rather than TB itself and the degree of immunosuppression is the most important predictor of survival in HIV-infected patients with tuberculosis.

CHALLENGES IN DIAGNOSING TB IN THE COINFECTED

Clinical Presentation

Active tuberculosis can occur at any CD4 cell count unlike most other opportunistic infections. However the clinical presentation is affected by the degree of immunosuppression. There is a bipolar pattern of clinical presentation of tuberculosis which is related to CD4 lymphocyte counts. In the early stages of immunosuppression, most persons with HIV infection present in the same fashion as others with tuberculosis who are not infected with HIV.

Early stage CD4 > 200 /mm^3: Typical presentation of upper lobe predominant cavitary pulmonary lesions such as cough, fever, weight loss and constitutional symptoms is seen. Some may present with unexplained dyspnea, chest pain or hemoptysis. Person living with HIV/AIDS should always be suspected of having tuberculosis when there is more than two weeks of cough which is usually productive in nature and/or fever lasting for more than two weeks.

Advance stage CD4 < 200/mm³: Atypical presentation with varied manifestations including extrapulmonary and disseminated TB is more common. However pulmonary disease remains the most common presentation even in advanced immunosuppression. Atypical manifestations like diffuse pulmonary involvement including the lower lobes with absence of cavitary lesions are seen more often. Extrapulmonary lesions such as hilar lymphadenopathy, pleural effusion, miliary TB, tubercular meningitis, cutaneous and chest wall abscess may also be seen.

The following conditions in a TB patient at the time of presentation or inspite of receiving Antitubercular drugs should arouse the suspicion of HIV infection:

- Oral/*Esophageal candidiasis*
- Chronic diarrhea more than one month
- Weight loss more than 10% in the last six month period
- Fever for more than one month
- *Herpes Zoster*
- Recurrent pneumonia
- Typhoid
- Oral hairy leukoplakia
- Present or past genital ulceration
- Kaposi's sarcoma
- Generalized dermatitis.

OTHER CONDITIONS MIMICKING PULMONARY TB IN THE HIV INFECTED

Due to the varied presentation of pulmonary tuberculosis in HIV infection, it is indeed a diagnostic challenge to distinguish it from other conditions with similar presentation of cough, fever, other chest sign and chest X-ray shadows. Acute bacterial pneumonia presents with a shorter history, commonest pathogen being *Streptococcus pneumoniae*. They respond well to standard treatment.

Diagnosing pulmonary kaposi sarcoma is difficult but it is usually associated with typical lesions on the skin or mucous membrane. The patient usually presents with cough, fever, hemoptysis, dyspnea or hemorrhagic pleural effusion.

Pneumocystis jirovecii pneumonia is far more common in HIV positive patients from the developed countries. It presents with a dry cough and fever which is associated with progressively increasing dyspnea resulting in oxygen desaturation and severe respiratory distress in some. Chest X-ray shows bilateral diffuse interstitial shadowing and definitive diagnosis is made on finding the cysts in induced sputum, bronchoalveolar lavage or biopsy specimen.

Other conditions which may mimic pulmonary tuberculosis are infections caused by nontuberculous mycobacteria such as *M. kansasii* and

M.avium complex, nocardiosis and certain fungal infections like cryptococcosis and histoplasmosis.

EXTRAPULMONARY TUBERCULOSIS

Extrapulmonary tuberculosis is more strongly HIV-related than pulmonary tuberculosis. In fact Mycobacteremia and extrapulmonary tuberculosis, especially meningitis and adenopathy, correlate with diminishing number of CD4 cells and degree of immunosuppression in the coinfected. HIV-related extrapulmonary tuberculosis is also a condition for WHO clinical stage 4 (advanced AIDS) diagnosis. Patients with HIV-related extrapulmonary tuberculosis often have disseminated disease and are at high risk of rapid clinical deterioration and death. In TB patient without HIV, extrapulmonary involvement is only seen in upto 15% cases where as it is commoner in those with HIV infection (20 to 50%). Many patients with extrapulmonary TB also have coexistent pulmonary TB and the clinician should always look out for the same.

TB lymphadenitis is the most common extrapulmonary TB. Cervical lymphadenopathy is the commonest site of presentation with the lymph nodes being usually large, bilateral, and asymmetrical. Usually they begin as firm discrete nodes which later on become fluctuant and matted. A few may be associated with skin breakdown with abscess and sinus formation which heal with scarring. The histological appearance of tuberculous lymph nodes from HIV positive patients depends on the degree of immunocompromise. Early in the disease there is caseating lesions with few or no AFB, but as immunity declines lymph nodes show little cellular reaction with many AFB. Some of this lymphadenopathy may also be caused by other nontuberculous mycobacteria such as *M. avium intracellulare.* Persistent generalized lymphadenopathy (PGL) is a feature of HIV infection which develops in upto 50% of HIV infected individuals. It is of no prognostic significance but is commonest differential diagnosis for TB lymphadenitis. The nodes are non-tender, symmetrical, and often involve the posterior cervical and epitrochlear nodes. PGL may slowly regress during the course of HIV infection and may disappear before the onset of AIDS. In populations with a high HIV prevalence, PGL is the commonest cause of lymphadenopathy.

Disseminated TB results from widespread blood borne spread of TB bacilli. Patients present with constitutional features rather than respiratory symptoms. They may have hepatosplenomegaly associated with fever of unknown origin and marked wasting. Commoner differential diagnosis includes the syndrome of HIV wasting disease ("slim disease") and bacteremia.

Tubercular pleural effusion is also commonly seen, which is usually unilateral and asymmetric and sometimes associated with pulmonary lesions as well. The presentation is usually with constitutional and local features like chest pain, breathlessness, tracheal and mediastinal shift away from the side of the effusion, decreased chest movement, dull percussion note and decreased breath sounds on the side of the effusion. Abdominal tuberculosis in HIV-infected patients is characterized by visceral lesions and intra-abdominal lymphadenopathy with necrosis, which is best visualized by computed tomography. Whereas, ascites and omental thickening are characteristic features in HIV-negative patients. Tubercular pericardial effusion and tubercular meningitis with focal brain lesions are the other common involvement in HIV patients.

Making an accurate diagnosis of extrapulmonary tuberculosis is far more complex and difficult than the usual smear positive pulmonary tuberculosis and a high index of clinical suspicion is necessary.

DRAWBACK OF SPUTUM MICROSCOPY

Sputum microscopy is the cornerstone of diagnosis of tuberculosis even in high HIV-prevalence areas. Patients suspected of having tuberculosis should have at least two sputum specimens examined for acid fast bacilli. HIV-infected, smear positive patients tend to excrete significantly fewer organisms per ml of sputum than HIV-negative patients, which can lead to AFB being missed if the appropriate number of sputum samples as well as adequate number of high power fields is not examined by microscopy. In early HIV infection, smear positive pulmonary tuberculosis is as common as in the non-HIV patients. The sputum negativity tends to increase as the HIV disease and immunosuppression progress. This is because cavitation is less likely in the coinfected with advanced immunosuppression. Cavitation is associated with increased numbers of extracellular acid-fast bacilli, thus a greater likelihood of a positive sputum smear in non-HIV infected patients with typical reactivation tuberculosis.

DILEMMA IN CHEST RADIOLOGY

Chest radiography is usually performed in cases suspected of being coinfected. However it has to be kept in mind that unlike the typical lesions seen in HIV negative tuberculosis patients such as unilateral or bilateral upper zone infiltrations or fluffy shadows with occasional calcification associated with single or multiple cavities, the patients with coinfection have various atypical radiographic features depending on degree of immunosuppression.

In HIV-infected patients with tuberculosis who have CD4 cell counts of 200 or more per cubic millimeter, chest radiographic findings include upper zone infiltrates and cavitation, findings similar to those in HIV-negative patients with tuberculosis. However, in HIV-infected patients with fewer than 200 CD4 cells per cubic millimeter, diffuse pulmonary infiltrates and patchy opacities usually involving more than one zone bilaterally without cavitation are the dominant radiological presentation on an X-ray chest. Lower lung field tuberculosis is also more prevalent in this group. Miliary or micronodular lesions, pleural effusion and mediastinal adenopathy is commonly seen, a situation similar to that in HIV-negative children with primary tuberculosis. Approximately 5% of HIV-infected patients with pulmonary tuberculosis have positive results on acid-fast staining of sputum, despite normal chest radiographs.

MANTOUX TEST

Though tuberculin test is frequently performed to determine infection with *Mycobacterium tuberculosis*, it is plagued by the drawbacks of high false positive rates and false negative rates especially due to anergy. Moreover it only tells about infection and is unable to distinguish it from active tubercular disease thereby decreasing its value as a tool for diagnosis in countries with high latent TB infection such as India.

Mantoux test determines the cellular immunity to tuberculin antigen and an induration of more than 5 mm to 1 Tuberculin Unit (TU) is considered to be a positive response in individuals with HIV infection. It has also been observed that many coinfected individuals with initial unresponsive Mantoux test become positive after being put on antiretroviral therapy, probably due to immune restoration. Thus the Mantoux test is positive in early disease whereas coinfected patients with advanced AIDS commonly have negative tuberculin-skin tests. Tuberculin reactivity of more than 10 mm is seen in up to 85% cases of pulmonary *tuberculosis* without HIV. Whereas it is positive in only 40 to 70% cases of TB in early HIV infection and barely in 10 to 30% cases with advanced HIV/AIDS.

TREATING HIV/TB COINFECTION

It is now comprehensively proven that both antituberculosis treatment (ATT) and highly active antiretroviral therapy (HAART) are indispensable in the management of patients with HIV/TB coinfection. HIV-positive TB patients have a much higher case-fatality during and after anti-TB treatment compared with HIV-negative patients. In Sub-Saharan Africa, up to 30% of HIV-positive smear-positive Pulmonary TB (PTB) patients die before the end of treatment. Evidence suggests that HIV-positive smear-negative PTB patients have a worse prognosis than those who have HIV-positive smear-positive PTB. Excess deaths in TB/HIV patients during and after treatment are partly due to TB itself and partly due to other HIV-related problems. These include septicemia, diarrhea, pneumonia, nontubercular mycobacterial infection, Kaposi's sarcoma, and cryptococcal meningitis. HAART not only reduces this increased mortality of HIV-infected patients with TB, which is significantly higher than that of HIV-negative TB patients but also reduces the risk of developing primary TB infection and reduces the risk of progression of latent infection to active tubercular disease. However there are significant pharmacokinetic interactions between the rifamycin component of antituberculosis treatment and antiretroviral drugs especially, protease inhibitors (PIs) and non-nucleoside reverse transcriptase inhibitors (NNRTIs).

The three principle issues regarding timing of co-treatment are:

1. Treatment of TB always takes precedence over the treatment of HIV infection
2. In patients who are already on HAART, the same has to be continued with appropriate modifications both in HAART and antituberculosis treatment
3. In patients who are not receiving HAART, the need and timing of initiation of HAART have to be decided after assessing the short-term risk of disease progression and death, based on CD4+ count and type of TB.

ANTITUBERCULAR TREATMENT

The antituberculosis treatment regimen in the HIV/TB coinfected is identical to those for HIV negative adults. Irrespective of HIV status, a new case of tuberculosis requires a minimum of six months of treatment with four standard drugs including INH (H), rifampicin (RIF), ethambutol (EMB) and pyrazinamide (PYZ) in the intensive phase and two drugs (H and RIF) in the continuation phase. This is the category one regimen of the Revised National Tuberculosis Control Program (RNTCP) followed in India. For patients with slow clinical response or extensive or disseminated disease, therapy is extended to nine months. Those coinfected patients with past history of relapse, default or failure of TB treatment receive an eight-month regimen. This regimen known as Cat II consists of two months of streptomycin with H, RIF, PYZ and EMB followed by one month of H, RIF, PYZ and EMB in the intensive phase. This is followed by five months of continuation phase consisting of H, RIF and EMB. It is only the category III regimen for patients with smear negative pulmonary TB and localized extrapulmonary TB consisting of four months of H, RIF and PYZ followed by two months of H and RIF, which is not recommended for HIV/TB coinfected patients. They should be put on Cat I instead. The thrice a week directly observed short course intermittent regimen (DOTS) is sufficiently effective in treating TB in the coinfected.

ANTIRETROVIRAL TREATMENT

Commonly used antiretroviral regimens usually consist of three or more drugs from two or three different classes of drugs. The three major classes of drugs are nucleoside reverse transcriptase inhibitors (NRTIs), non-nucleoside reverse transcriptase inhibitors (NNRTIs) and protease inhibitors (PIs) **(Table 33.1)**.

Table 33.1: Antiretroviral drugs

Drug	*Dose*	*Side effects*
	NRTI	
Zidovudine (ZDV)	300 mg twice daily	Anemia, agranulocytosis
Stavudine (d4T)	40 mg twice daily	neuropathy, pancreatitis
Lamivudine (3TC)	150 mg twice daily	nausea, headache agranulocytosis
Abacavir (ABC)	300 mg twice daily	sleep disturbance, hypersensitivity
	NNRTI	
Efavirenz (EFZ)	600 mg once daily	Skin rash, hepatitis, neuropsychiatric disturbances (with EFZ)
Nevirapine (NVP)	200 mg twice daily	
	PI	
Nelfinavir (NFV)	1250 mg twice daily	• Elevated serum cholesterol,
Indinavir/ritonavir (IDV/r)	800 mg/100 mg twice daily	triglycerides and blood glucose
Saquinavir/ritonavir (SQV/r)	1000 mg/100 mg twice daily	• Nausea • Diarrhea
Lopinavir/ritonavir (LPV/r)	400 mg/100 mg twice daily	• Kidney stones (with IDV)

Drug-Drug Interaction

Two of these classes, NNRTIs and PIs, have clinically relevant drug interactions with the rifamycins. The key locus of the drug-drug interactions is the cytochrome P450-3A system in the intestinal wall and the liver. The rifamycins are inducers of this system, thereby decreasing the serum concentrations of drugs metabolized by this enzyme system. Rifampicin is the most potent, and rifabutin is the least potent inducer. The protease inhibitors and the non-nucleoside reverse transcriptase inhibitors are metabolized by CYP3A, and therefore may be affected by the rifamycins. For example, rifampicin reduces levels of protease inhibitors (except ritonavir) by 75 to 95%. This would lead to markedly decreased antiviral activity and more rapid emergence of protease inhibitor resistance. Hence, protease inhibitors (except ritonavir) cannot be used with rifampicin. Similarly the level of nevirapine, an NNRTI also falls drastically, making it unreliable when co-prescribed with rifampicin.

Since, rifamycins are the most potent antitubercular drug especially against the slow growing bacilli, it is recommended to include them in any antitubercular regimen being given to the coinfected patient.

Recommended Regimen of Highly Active Antiretroviral Therapy in TB Patients

HAART refers to the use of a combination of at least three antiretroviral (ART) drugs to form a maximally suppressive regimen. In India, the National AIDS Control Organization recommends that the coinfected patients should receive an efavirenz (EFZ) based regimen as the first line therapy.

- First line therapy (2NRTI + 1NNRTI) available in the national program for the coinfected:
  - Zidovudine + Lamivudine + Efavirenz
  - Stavudine + Lamivudine + Efavirenz
- Alternative first-line treatment regimen (Triple NRTI containing Abacavir)
- Reserve/2nd line treatment regimen (Regimen consisting of Protease Inhibitor + 2 NRTI, to be used when first line treatment fails).

When to Start HAART in the Coinfected (Table 33.2)

Table 33.2: Starting HAART

CD4 Count	*Starting HAART in relation to antituberculous treatment (ATT)*
Count not available	Between **two and eight weeks**. HAART should be started as soon as TB treatment is tolerated
CD4 **<200 cells**/cu.mm.	**After eight weeks**
CD4 between 200 and 350 cells/cu.mm	Defer HAART and re-evaluate patient at eight weeks and at the end of TB treatment
CD4 >350 cells/cu.mm	

OVERLAPPING DRUG TOXICITY

Drug toxicity is a major challenge when multidrug therapy is required for any medical condition. It is more common in patients receiving both anti-tubercular and antiretroviral therapies. This is because concurrent therapy of coinfection requires concomitant administration of at least four different antituberculosis agents and at least three antiretroviral drugs. This risk increases with advanced immunosuppression and occurs usually in first two months of treatment when the patient should be carefully monitored. Only serious or life-threatening side effects, which are less frequent requires discontinuation of therapy and most cases can be managed symptomatically.

Almost all drugs used have varying degrees of hepatotoxicity, however special care need to be taken when rifampicin and pyrazinamide is combined with the nucleoside reverse transcription inhibitors or nevirapine. Isoniazid induced peripheral neuropathy is more common in HIV patients on antiretroviral therapy and pyridoxine must be added to the treatment regimen. Antitubercular drug thiacetazone should never be prescribed in HIV patients due to the very high risk of developing Steven Johnson Syndrome. Other skin manifestations are seen when ATT is given with non-nucleoside reverse transcriptase inhibitor (NNRTIs) or protease inhibitors (PIs).

Rifampicin reduces the effectiveness of oral contraceptives and an alternate means of contraception must be used. Drug toxicity has been implicated as a major cause of discontinuation of antiretroviral therapy and of interruptions of TB and/or HIV therapy during concurrent treatment of coinfection.

IMMUNE RECONSTITUTION INFLAMMATORY SYNDROME

Immune reconstitution inflammatory syndrome (IRIS) or paradoxical reactions are defined as transient worsening or appearance of new signs, symptoms, or radiographic manifestations of tuberculosis that occur after initiation of antiretroviral treatment and are not the result of treatment failure or a second process. The paradoxical reactions in HIV-infected patients are due to restoration of immunity toward mycobacterial antigens released as tubercle bacilli are killed by antitubercular therapy. It is associated with substantial reduction in viral load and increase in CD4 count. Paradoxical reaction can be demonstrated by marked increase in delayed type hypersensitivity reaction such as tuberculin skin testing.

Risk factors include early initiation of antiretroviral therapy, i.e. within two months of starting antitubercular treatment, low CD4 count, presence of extrapulmonary and disseminated TB and high viral load. Such reactions occur within days to weeks after starting antiretroviral therapy and are mostly self limiting. It is seen in up to 36% of coinfected patients, and generally lasts for 10 to 40 days.

Though patient may show widely varied manifestation ranging from mild fever to sudden appearance of acute respiratory failure, the common presentations include fever, increased or initial appearance of adenopathy, new or worsening pulmonary infiltrates, serositis like pleural effusion or ascites, cutaneous lesions, and new or expanding central nervous system mass lesions. The differential diagnoses include treatment failure, progression of TB, drug hypersensitivity and other infections common among immunocompromised patients.

Most cases respond to symptomatic treatment with nonsteroidal anti-inflammatory drugs (NSAIDs) along with antiretroviral therapy. Oral corticosteroids for four to six weeks may be necessary in severe and life threatening situations or when there is no adequate response to NSAIDs. There may be a rare need to stop antiretroviral therapy.

ROLE OF CORTICOSTEROIDS IN HIV-TB COINFECTION

Steroids may depress immunity and increase risk of opportunistic infections in HIV-positive patients. There exists no clear guideline regarding regular corticosteroid use in HIV-TB coinfection. However in certain life-threatening circumstances adjuvant steroid therapy may be of benefit in the coinfected patients. Steroids are recommended in HIV positive patients with pericardial TB. They may also be of use in TB meningitis with decreased consciousness, neurological defects or spinal block, TB of adrenal glands, TB laryngitis with life-threatening airway obstruction, massive tubercular lymph node enlargement with pressure effects and in treatment of paradoxical reactions.

MULTIDRUG RESISTANT TB AND HIV COINFECTION

People living with HIV/AIDS have a far greater risk of acquiring drug resistance due to many factors. Malabsorption of antitubercular drugs especially of rifampicin is known to occur in HIV patients. Rifampicin mono-resistance is more common in HIV infected patients, the reason of which is not yet clear. Increased drug resistence is also due to decreased immunity and the inability to eliminate the tubercle bacilli in the HIV positive patients. Increased opportunity to acquire the infection due to overcrowding, exposure to patients with MDR-TB due to increased hospital visits is also seen. MDR-TB is defined as tuberculosis caused by *Mycobacterium tuberculosis* which is resistant to at least isoniazid and rifampicin. The prognosis of HIV/MDR-TB coinfected is very poor and the treatment is for at least 24 months. Treatment includes six to nine months of intensive phase consisting of at least six drugs such as kanamycin injection, ethionamide, cycloserine, a flouroquinolone, pyrazinamide and ethambutol. This is followed by the continuation phase of 18 months of ethionamide, cycloserine, a flouroquinolone and ethambutol.

CHEMOPROPHYLACTIC TREATMENT

Use of preventive therapy for Latent TB infection (LTBI) in HIV patients has shown significant decrease in incidence of developing active tuberculosis as well as mortality. It is recommended that all HIV cases with Mantoux test of 5 mm or more should be given chemoprophylaxis of Isoniazid of 6 to 12 months. Role of lifelong isoniazid is presently being evaluated. Shorter regimens are also available, such as two months of rifampicin and pyrazinamide but they are likely to have more drug toxicity. It is very important to reliably rule out active TB before starting the prophylactic treatment, especially in countries where TB is endemic. Co-trimoxazole prophylaxis is also routinely recommended in the coinfected patients.

BCG Vaccination

WHO recommends that in countries where risk of TB is high, asymptomatic HIV infected children should receive BCG vaccination at the earliest as per the immunization policy. It is however contraindicated in a child having symptomatic HIV disease. BCG, which is a live attenuated bacilli, when given to a symptomatic HIV positive individual may lead to disseminated BCG disease. Disseminated BCG disease is very rare and is treated with isoniazid and rifampicin given together.

JOINT HIV/TB ACTION PLAN

In India the Revised National TB Control Program (RNTCP) and National AIDS Control Organization (NACO) have decided to coordinate with each other to promote early diagnosis and treatment of both HIV and TB. This involves coordination of service delivery and cross-referrals, where all diagnosed TB patients at the Designated Microcopy Center (DMC) of the RNTCP will be referred for voluntary HIV testing. Similarly all clients at the Integrated Counseling and Testing Center (ICTC) of the NACO, who are symptomatic of TB will be referred to the nearest DMC for further evaluation. Joint training programs for service providers involved in RNTCP and NACO have also been planned.

CONCLUSION

The duel epidemic of HIV/TB has worked synergistically to overwhelm the TB control program of many nations. Tuberculosis accelerates the progression of HIV infection and HIV increases the likelihood of active TB disease. The coinfection also makes diagnosing TB a challenge because it alters the clinical, radiological and microbiological picture with varied atypical presentations.

However, there is no difference in the TB treatment in the coinfected, and the existing regimens are quite effective as well. Co-treatment with HAART and rifampicin containing ATT given Directly Observed (via DOTS) has significantly improved the scenario in these coinfected patients. But prescribing HAART and ATT together have generated new complex issues of overlapping drug toxicity, complex drug-drug interaction, paradoxical reactions and difficulty in maintaining patient compliance and adherence to treatment. However, priority should remain to detect cases of TB early and treat them adequately in both HIV positive as well as negative patients to substantially reduce disease transmission in countries with high tuberculosis prevalence. Thus a strong coordination between the national TB program and the AIDS control program is required for effective management of HIV-TB patients.

BIBLIOGRAPHY

1. A guide to monitoring and evaluation for collaborative TB/HIV activities, WHO 2004.
2. Guidelines for implementing collaborative TB and HIV programme activities, WHO 2003.
3. Improving the diagnosis and treatment of smear-negative pulmonary and extrapulmonary tuberculosis among adults and adolescents. Recommendations for HIV-prevalent and resource-constrained settings, WHO 2006.
4. TB/HIV, A Clinical Manual, WHO 2004.

34 Chapter Sexually Transmitted Diseases in India: Historical Aspects and Emerging Trends (Except HIV Infection)

DM Thappa

INTRODUCTION

The older terminology of "venereal diseases" (VDs) largely has been superseded in the past 50 years by "sexually transmitted diseases" (STDs), and more recently by "sexually transmitted infections" (STIs). To some, venereal diseases came to be viewed as a narrow and pejorative term limited to gonorrhea, syphilis, chancroid, lymphogranuloma venereum, and granuloma inguinale, and related VD control laws. The term sexually transmitted diseases more easily incorporate the many newly discovered sexually transmitted agents and syndromes. Sexually transmitted diseases (STDs) include diseases that are transmitted by sexual intercourse. Sexual transmission requires the agent to be present in one partner, the other partner to be susceptible to infection with that agent and that the sex partners engage in sexual practices which can transmit the pathogen. Sexually transmitted infection (STI) differs from sexually transmitted disease (STD) in that STD conventionally includes infections resulting in clinical diseases that may involve the genitalia and other parts of the body participating in sexual interaction e.g., syphilis, gonorrhea, chancroid, donovanosis, nongonococcal urethritis, genital warts, herpes genitalis etc. STI in addition, includes infections that may not cause clinical disease of genitals, but are transmitted by sexual interaction e.g., all STDs and hepatitis B, HIV and HTLV-1 infections. Now-a-days, the term STI is preferred, since it covers all the diseases that can be transmitted by sexual intercourse. However, for all practical purposes, both STI and STD are used synonymously.

Venereology (the study of venereal diseases) today encompasses more than the five classical venereal diseases (syphilis, gonorrhea, chancroid, donovanosis and lymphogranuloma venereum). A growing number of other diseases are being identified that might be considered the new generation of sexually transmitted diseases (STDs). Their importance is newly recognized due to the development of laboratory techniques of diagnosis and increasing awareness of the consequences of STDs in areas of health and society.

Origin of STDs

Origin of venereal (sexually transmitted) diseases is obscure. Medical historians and other historians have often suggested that well-known diseases such as syphilis, gonorrhea, chancroid and lymphogranuloma venereum have existed since earliest times. This may or may not be true and some of these individuals may have drawn conclusions from ancient texts and manuscripts that may not be accurate. While the infections certainly exist in *Homo sapiens*, did they occur in the preceding species *Homo erectus* prior to 150,000 BC? No one knows, but the French philosopher Voltaire summed it up well when he declared in his *Dictionnaire philosophique* that venereal diseases are like the fine arts - it is pointless to ask who invented them.

Among the uneducated and uninformed people in India, we often hear remarks to the effect that the occurrence of venereal disease is a 'visitation from God,' 'a sign of growing adolescence,' 'a sign of maturity,' 'the result of eating nettle leaves' and 'from sexual intercourse with menstruating woman'. Such fallacious ideas about the causation of venereal diseases are still prevalent all over the world with varying emphasis. In the field of medicine, the ancient Hindus carried their researches farther than any of their contemporaries. The Upanishads contain the most convincing evidence of their passion for enquiry into the nature of things. Padmini, or the Lotus woman, is the symbol of woman beauty in Hindu literature. According to Hindu mythology, in the beginning, the Lord of Beings (Brahma) created men and women and laid down rules for regulating their existence with regard to *Dharma* (acquisition of religious merit), *Artha* (acquisition of wealth, property, etc.) and *Kama* (love, pleasure and sensual gratification). The commandments related to *Kama* were expounded by Nandi, the follower of Mahadeva. This document written by Nandi, known as Kama Sutra (aphorisms on love), was transformed into a small volume of Sanskrit literature by Vatsyayana between the 1st and 6th century of the Christian era. This manuscript is known by the name of Vatsyayana Kama Sutra. This document was withheld from public gaze as sex was considered a taboo amongst Hindus. This Sanskrit document was later translated into English by Sir Richard Burton and FF Arbuthanot and was published in England in 1883. There is no mention of venereology in the days of Kama Sutra.

Syphilis

In the past, some attempts have been made to identify syphilis and gonorrhea in ancient Hindu (Ayurvedic) texts, but evidence strongly suggests that syphilis, at least, was unknown in India before the early 16th century. So explosive was the nature of epidemic in this region during that time and so deep was the cultural and national impact that various religious/cultural communities started blaming each other as the source. Careful examination of available records shows that Charaka and Sushruta, two ancient ayurvedic physicians, did not know anything about syphilis. However, Bloomfield, Hirsch, Hessler and other Orientalists have suggested that syphilis was prevalent in ancient India. Some of the first references to the disease and its treatment are to be found in the *Bhavaprakasa,* a mid-sixteenth-century text, reputedly the work of Bhavamisra, an Ayurvedic physician at Benares. During that period and subsequently for a long time, syphilis was known in India as the Portuguese disease, or *firanga* or *firangi roga,* terms that identified it with the *firangis* ('Franks'), or Europeans. According to historians, the disease was first recognized in India in 1498 after the arrival of Vasco de Gama, who had left Portugal in 1497. It seems probable that the Portuguese introduced the disease to India from Europe in the early 16th century. The researches of Okamura in Japan, Susuki in China and Jolly and others in India show that syphilis was introduced into this country from Europe. By the early 19th century, when the British had gained ascendancy over a large part of the subcontinent, syphilis was already widely disseminated, though the extent of its incidence can only be guessed at.

Gonorrhea

Authentic records of gonorrhea in India can only be found during the British Empire in India. During British Raj, in official statistics of the army, venereal diseases like syphilis, gonorrhea and soft chancre (now called as chancroid) figured. In regiments of the British army stationed in India, the percentage of troops admitted to hospital with venereal diseases (identified in almost equal proportion as primary syphilis and gonorrhea) rose to 205 per 1,000 in 1875 and peaked at 522 per 1,000 in 1895. For unexplained reasons, syphilis was relatively more common and gonorrhea less common in the army personnel of Indian origin than in the British army in India.

Chancroid

Chancroid, one of the five classic venereal diseases, was first described by Brassereau in 1852 in France. The venereal diseases in the British Army were regarded as comprising of syphilis, gonorrhea and soft chancre, but it was decided to ignore the last named as not of public health importance in the run-up to the Royal Commission of 1916. In the Army in India (71,001 men), the venereal disease rate in the year 1912 was 55.5 per 1,000 (10.1% of all admissions). In the army at home, in India, the total venereal disease rate of 56.5 per 1,000 consisted of 18.7 for primary and secondary syphilis, 29.5 for gonorrhea and 8.3 for soft sore.

Donovanosis

Historically, donovanosis, formerly called as granuloma inguinale, was first recognized and described in India. It was first described in 1881 in Madras, India, under the name of 'serpiginous ulcer' by Kenneth MacLeod, a Scot, who joined the Indian Medical Service and became professor of surgery in Calcutta. Cause of it was found by Colonel Charles Donovan. In 1905, he described the intracellular bodies, which bear his name and was the co-discoverer of the etiological agent in kala-azar. So-called 'Donovan bodies' were found in the exudate from an oral lesion of the disease in a ward boy of General Hospital in Madras. The nature of these was disputed from the beginning. Donovan himself thought that they were protozoa. It was not until 1943 that it was clearly shown that the 'Donovan bodies' were bacterial in nature. The natural history of donovanosis and its probable venereal nature was subsequently elucidated by others.

Lymphogranuloma Venereum

In 1902, Caddy was the first to record cases of lymphogranuloma venereum (LGV) in India under the title 'Climatic bubo'. At the Institute of Venereology in Madras, 3,884 cases of LGV were diagnosed between 1968 and 1977, accounting for 6% of STD cases seen in the same period. Towards the end of the 19th century, most authors in India held the opinion that disease was due to climatic influences (mainly tropical) and consequently, many textbooks today still refer to LGV as 'Climatic bubo'.

Other STDs

However, no description of genital warts, herpes genitalis and trichomoniasis is found in the comparatively modern Indian literature of the early 20th century. Despite considerable doubt by most observers, by 1920s and 1930s many venereologists had concluded that genital warts are sexually transmitted diseases. Genital herpes was rarely considered in the differential diagnosis of genital ulcers prior to 1965. It was only in 1966 that herpes genitalis was recognized as a venereal disease. At present, it is the most common STD in some of the STD clinics in India. Donne first described the protozoal organism *Trichomonas vaginalis* in 1836, which he observed in purulent genital secretions from both men and women. Microbiological investigations of chlamydial infections began in 1907 when Halberstaedter and Prowazek detected intracytoplasmic chlamydial inclusions in the conjunctival scrapings of nonhuman primates that were experimentally infected with material collected from the conjunctiva of patients with active trachoma. Similar inclusions were later demonstrated in conjunctival cells of trachomatous patients, in scrapings from the conjunctiva of the eyes of babies with ophthalmia neonatorum, from the endocervix of mothers of these babies and from the urethra of patients with bacterial urethritis. In a study published in 2000, among 319 women with vaginal discharge attending a reproductive health clinic in New Delhi, India, the most common infection was bacterial vaginosis (26%). At least one sexually transmitted infection was detected in 21.9% of women. The prevalence of C. *trachomatis* infection was 12.2%, *trichomoniasis* 10% and syphilis 2.2%.

Changing Trends of STDs/STIs

Sexually transmitted infections (STIs) are more dynamic than other diseases prevailing in the community. Their epidemiological profile varies from country to country and from one region to another within a country, depending upon ethnographic, demographic, socio-economic and health factors. The clinical pattern is also a result of the interaction among pathogens, the behaviors that transmit them and the effectiveness of preventive and control interventions.

Global Trends of STDs

Sexually transmitted diseases (STDs) remain a major public health challenge in the United States. While substantial progress has been made in preventing, diagnosing, and treating certain STDs in recent years, CDC estimates that 19 million new infections occur each year, almost half of them among young people aged 15 to 24. Chlamydia remains the most commonly reported infectious disease in the United States. It is estimated that there are approximately 2.8 million new cases of chlamydia in the United States each year. The increases in reported cases and rates reflect the continued expansion of screening efforts and increased use of more sensitive diagnostic tests; however, this trend may also reflect an actual increase in infections. Women, especially young women, are hit hardest by Chlamydia and the long-term consequences of untreated disease are much more severe for women.

Gonorrhea is the second most commonly reported infectious disease in the United States. Following a 74% decline in the rate of reported gonorrhea from 1975 through 1997, overall gonorrhea rates appear to have reached a plateau in recent years. Like chlamydia, however, gonorrhea is substantially under-diagnosed and under-reported, and approximately twice as many new infections are estimated to occur each year as are reported. African Americans remain the group most heavily affected by gonorrhea, with a rate in 2005 that was 18 times greater than the rate for whites. Ethnic minorities in the United States have traditionally had higher rates of reported gonorrhea and other STDs, which reflects limited access to quality health care, poverty, and higher prevalence of disease in these populations.

The rate of primary and secondary syphilis—the most infectious stages of the disease—decreased throughout the 1990s, and in 2000 reached an all-time low. However, over the past five years, the syphilis rate in the United States has been increasing. Between 2004 and 2005, the national syphilis rate increased 11.1 percent, from 2.7 to 3.0 cases per 100,000 populations. The syphilis rate among men is now nearly six times the rate among women, whereas the rates were almost equivalent a decade ago. Additionally, prior CDC research has estimated that more than half of syphilis cases in recent years have occurred among men who have sex with men (MSM). Although wide disparities persist, racial gaps in syphilis rates are narrowing. While syphilis rates remained substantially lower among females than males, rates among females increased for the first time in over a decade, with an increase of 12.5 percent from 2004 to 2005.

In Europe, data on Chlamydia often reflects testing patterns and not true incidence rates. It is primarily transmitted among young people and is probably the most common STD all over Europe. Estimates indicate that 70 to 75% of women infected with Chlamydia trachomatis are symptom-free.

Like chlamydia infection, gonorrhea also often goes undetected, especially in women. Significant decreases in the incidence of gonorrhea have been noted in all regions of Europe since 1980, and the disease is now mainly seen in young homosexual men, highly sexually active individuals and socio-economically deprived communities. In the last 8 to 10 years, a parallel trend has been noted for gonorrhea and HIV infection, reflecting a common mode of transmission, and similar risk groups for both infections.

The incidence of syphilis decreased dramatically during the 1980s, stabilized in the 1990s, and has recently increased since 1999/2000. This increased incidence may be attributable to better surveillance systems and case detection. Episodic outbreaks of syphilis occur in certain high risk populations, such as men who have sex with men (MSM), commercial sex workers and drug users.

Very few European countries routinely collect data on herpes simplex and human papilloma virus infections. Of the countries that report to the WHO, high levels of incidence (20-70/100 000) have been reported over the last five years in the United Kingdom and the Russian federation, among others. The highest levels of HPV infection have been reported in the United Kingdom (80-120/100000) and Ireland (100/100000) in 2000. Recently, several outbreaks of lymphogranuloma venereum have been noted in several countries, including Europe, the United States and Canada. It is primarily reported in MSM, among whom the majority is HIV positive.

Current Status of STDs in India

Sexually transmitted diseases (STDs) constitute a major public health problem for both developing and developed countries. The emergence of human immunodeficiency virus (HIV) infection has increased the importance of measures aimed at control of STDs. A proper understanding of the patterns of STDs prevailing in different geographic regions of a country is necessary for proper planning and implementation of STD control strategies. It is with this aim that the author has reviewed the past 25 year relevant published literature from India.

In the year 1987, a retrospective, data analysis of sexually transmitted diseases was carried out to study the pattern of these diseases in a tertiary care center in Chandigarh. One thousand five hundred and seventy one patients were seen from January 1977 to October 1985. Males constituted 95.5% of this group and females the remaining 4.5%. Commonest age group affected was 20 to 29 years in both sexes. Condyloma acuminata was the commonest STD (21.40%), followed by gonorrhea (16.9%), chancroid (12.2%), genital herpes (11.4%), syphilis (10.4%), non specific ulcers (7.1%), donovanosis (6.3%), mixed infections (5.3%) and non-specific urethritis (NSU) (4.1%). What was obvious from this study is that viral STDs have started showing their dominance in otherwise dominant bacterial STD scenario. But if we look at the scenario of STDs in and around Udaipur, the relative incidence of chancroid was found to be higher (37.7%) than syphilis (32.4%), followed by gonorrhea (24.7%) mixed infections (3.38%), donovanosis (1.1%) and lymphogranuloma venereum (0.3%) among 1093 STD cases attending this clinic in the past 10 years. Here, bacterial STDs were still common.

Moving on to another state, at Cuttack in Orissa, 516 patients with STD were analyzed during the period 1993 to 1994. Herpes genitalis (21.89%) was found to be commonest STD followed by syphilis (16.27%), chancroid (11.82%) and granuloma inguinale (7.55%), gonococcal urethritis and genital warts (3.87% each). LGV was found in 0.58% of cases, HIV infection in three cases only (0.56%). Other miscellaneous infections like candidiasis (13.75%), trichomoniasis (2.7%) and molluscum (2.14%) were responsible in 18% as a whole and nonspecific infection in 14%. Look at the trends of STDs at Vadodara, Gujarat and they seem to be similar to that recorded at Cuttack. In the year 1995 to 96, 460 (2.45%) STD cases were recorded in this center. Frequency of different STDs observed in descending order was herpes genitalis (28.82%), gonorrhea (8.26%), granuloma inguinale (0.43%), and genital wart (8.9%). Other miscellaneous infections like candidiasis, trichomoniasis and molluscum constituted 18.47%. No HIV case was detected.

The relation between sexually transmitted diseases (STDs) and risk of HIV infection has been a subject of increasing interest. Hence, a study was conducted in the STD clinic of the department of dermatology and STD, JIPMER, Pondicherry, south India, between January 1993 and December 1997, to estimate the incidence of different STDs and frequency of HIV seropositivity among various STDs. The patients were from neighboring Tamil Nadu state and Pondicherry itself. The study group consisted of all new consecutive STD cases having high risk behavior and/or having present or past history of STDs, irrespective of their age and sex. Out of the

1110 patients recorded, 168 were seropositive for HIV, giving a prevalence rate of 15.14%. Annual breakdown revealed an upward trend from 8.6% in 1993 to 23.52% in 1997. The mean age of the group was 29.8 years, with a male to female ratio of 3.63:1. When the STDs were broadly classified into ulcerative and non-ulcerative groups, the prevalence of HIV was much higher in the group with ulcerative STDs (17.1%) than those with non-ulcerative STDs (9.5%). Genital herpes was the commonest STD followed by syphilis, condyloma acuminata, and others; 9.4% of the patients had concurrent infection with more than one STD.

A retrospective data analysis of one thousand STD patients from 1994 to 1998 at Medical College, Trivandrum was carried out. Males constituted 61.1% and females 38.9% in the study. The commonest STD was syphilis, both in men and women followed by herpes genitalis and condylomata acuminata. The prevalence of herpes genitalis and condylomata acuminata showed an increase with a definite decline in the prevalence of gonorrhea. HIV was detected in 3.2% of the patients.

A retrospective data analysis was carried out to find the trends in frequency and distribution of different STDs in North Eastern (NE) India during 1995 to 1999. The commonest STD was chancroid (25.7%) followed by condylomata acuminata (CA), nongonococcal urethritis (NGU), lymphogranuloma venereum (LGV), syphilis, gonorrhea (GONO), herpes genitalis (HG), mixed infection (MI) and balanoposthitis (BP). HIV infection accounted for 9.62% of the total STD patients. A comparison of the present data with that reported a decade back (1986 - 1990) revealed a sharp decline in the incidence of syphilis, chancroid, GONO, whereas a conspicuous upward trend in CA and NGU was noticed. Similarly, a retrospective study was undertaken from the year 1988 to 1998 to study the pattern of sexually transmitted diseases in and around Lucknow. Among 1890 patients examined, chancroid predominated followed by syphilis, gonorrhea, genital warts, herpes genitalis, LGV and non-specific urethritis. The incidence of donovanosis was the lowest.

In a recently published study, data of 686 patients with STDs was studied to find the pattern of STDs and to analyze the changes during a ten-year period from 1990 among patients attending Medical College Hospital, Kottayam. There were 504 males and 182 females in the total of 686 patients. Marital contact alone was reported by 123 (67.6%) female patients. Genital ulcer diseases (GUDs) accounted for the maximum number of STDs, with 504 cases (73.5%), followed by condylomata acuminata (17.5%) and gonorrhea (10.1%). Forty-three patients had multiple infections. The total number of patients during the first year of study was 129, while it was 41 during the last year. Bacterial STDs showed a striking reduction in numbers. The decline was less marked in the case of viral STDs.

Changing trends of the profile of STIs and HIV seropositivity in STD clinic attendees over a 15 year period at a regional STD center in New Delhi were analyzed. The STI profile and HIV seropositivity were compared between 1990 to 1993 (A), 1994 to 1997 (B), 1998 to 2001 (C) and 2002 to 2004 (D). Antimicrobial resistance pattern of *N. gonorrhoeae* was determined by standard techniques and compared between the last three periods. Of the 78,617 STD attendees, 12,709 (16.2%) had STIs. During period A, genital discharges and during B, C and D, genital ulcerative diseases were predominant. Syphilis was the commonest STI. There was significant rise in the cases of syphilis, herpes genitalis and genital warts and reduction in that of chancroid, lymphogranuloma venereum (LGV), donovanosis, candidiasis, trichomoniasis and bacterial vaginosis cases. The number of cases with primary syphilis diminished significantly ($P<0.001$), with a concomitant rise in secondary and early latent syphilis. A rising trend was observed in the HIV seropositivity during the different periods. The association of HIV seropositivity was consistently more in patients presenting with genital ulcers specially syphilis, and rose significantly from A (0.6%) to C (8.8%), but became stationary during D. A drastic change in the antimicrobial resistance of *N. gonorrhoeae* from B to C and C to D and the emergence of less sensitive isolates to ceftriaxone during the later part of the study were observed.

Sharma and Khandpur reviewed the changing patterns of different STIs (excluding HIV infection) in India and their various risk factors. It was observed that most of the published data are institution based. There is a paucity of community-based data, except for information obtained from high risk groups such as commercial sex workers, truck drivers, hotel workers and drug abusers. From the literature search undertaken, it was observed that during the 1960s and 1970s, bacterial infections including syphilis, chancroid and gonorrhea were the major STIs, while viral infections caused by herpes simplex virus and human papillomavirus were so rare that they merited publication as case reports. As in developed countries, there has been a rise in viral and chlamydial infections and a relative fall in the incidence of traditional infections.

To sum up, bacterial STDs like chancroid and gonorrhea are showing a declining trend, but the viral STDs like herpes genitalis and condylomata acuminata are showing upward trend. There is a decline in the number of patients with STDs attending the hospital. Whether this is due to an actual decrease in the incidence of STDs or due to other factors is uncertain. The increased availability of facilities for treatment of STDs at peripheral centers might be a factor leading to a decline in the number of patients with STDs approaching higher centers like the teaching hospital where this study was undertaken. The emphasis on the syndromic approach to the management of STDs might have increased the accessibility to healthcare for these patients with STDs. Awareness about HIV and fear of contracting the STDs are likely to have influenced the risk-taking behavior of people, thereby reducing the likelihood of being infected with STDs. Another factor to be considered is the widespread use of antibacterials, including quinolones and the new macrolides, for the treatment of other diseases. This can result in partial treatment or modified course of the bacterial STDs, thereby leading to apparent reduction in the total number of cases of STDs attending STD clinics as well as a decrease in the proportion of bacterial to viral STDs. The evident decline of the bacterial STDs with an apparent increase of the viral STDs is the trend worth noting. A word of caution need to be exercised in the interpretation of the above data which is institution or tertiary care center based, hence many of changing patterns of STIs may not be true. Readers may use their expertise in interpretation of this data.

Emerging STI Scenario

With regard to India, most STIs are managed in the informal and private medical sectors or are self treated. STIs survey data are limited in India, but these surveys indicate a very diverse picture. In community-based surveys of married and unmarried women in India, the chlamydia prevalence ranged between 0.5% and 28.7%, gonorrhea between 0% and 4.2% and syphilis between 0.2% and 10.5%. During the last 10 to 15 years, after the emergence of AIDS and owing mainly to fear of AIDS, rates of gonorrhea, syphilis, hepatitis B infection and HIV have declined by 80 to 95% or more in the USA. For the past 7 to 9 years, STI rates in homosexual men again are rising modestly. Globally, the HIV incidence is still rising in some areas of Africa, Asia and Eastern Europe and declining in others. In India, the main strategy aimed at achieving effective management for people with established infections has been to integrate STD services into the existing health care system, with special emphasis on integration at the primary health care (PHC) level. The National AIDS Control Organization (NACO) for case management at this level recommends syndromic management. Effectiveness of syndromic management in women is currently under debate. The NACO is now also focusing on women reproductive health issues and involving gynecologists.

Future Directions

Donovanosis will be eradicated in several nations; but syphilis eradication will only be successful by 2020. Gonorrhea, chlamydia, chancroid and trichomoniasis may also persist despite their curability. With the exception of hepatitis B, HIV and other blood borne pathogens will continue to flourish until blood supplies and medical injections as well as illicit drug use and tattooing are made safe. Genitoanal warts and herpes will also persist and possibly increase, as may candidiasis, vulvovaginitis, bacterial vaginosis, balanitis, prostatitis. The problems of spreading HIV epidemic, drug resistance, poor health facilities, and financial constraints are definitely a great hindrance in achieving the desired reduction in the incidence and prevalence of STIs. In India, the main strategy aimed at achieving effective management for people with established infections has been to integrate STD services into the existing health care system, with a special emphasis on integration at the primary health care (PHC) level. Syndromic management is recommended by the National AIDS Control Organization (NACO) for case management at this level. The effectiveness of syndromic management in women is currently under debate. The NACO is now also focusing on women reproductive health issues and involving gynecologists.

Vast numbers of people in India are severely disadvantaged in terms of income, education, power structures, and gender. Addressing these basic issues of human rights lies at the core of achieving better health outcomes (including reproductive and infectious diseases) in India. Such a challenge is formidable in terms of its required scope and coverage, but lies at the heart of improving sexual health for the greatest number of people in India.

BIBLIOGRAPHY

1. Sharma VK, Khandpur S. Changing patterns of sexually transmitted infections in India. Natl Med J India 2004;17(6):310-9.
2. Thappa DM, Kaimal S. Sexually transmitted infections in India: Current status (except human immunodeficiency virus/acquired immunodeficiency syndrome). Indian J Dermatol 2007;52:78-82.
3. Thappa DM. Historical aspects of sexually transmitted diseases and AIDS. In: Sharma VK (Ed). Sexually Transmitted Diseases and AIDS, 2nd edn. New Delhi: Viva Books 2009.pp.69-87.
4. World Health Organization (homepage on the internet). Trends in sexually transmitted infections and HIV in the European region, 1980-2005. Technical briefing document 01B/06 Copenhagen, 12 September 2006. Available from: www.euro.who.int/Document/RC56/etb01b.pdf.

Section C

Appendices

Appendices

Appendix 1

Important Events in the History of Communicable Diseases

Year	Event
1850	Confusion between typhoid and typhus fever (caused by *Salmonella*) was resolved with publication in 1850 of Willam Jenner's book—Identity and nonidentity of Typhoid and Typhus fever.
1854	Outbreak of cholera stopped in London when Dr John snow tied the handle of the Broak street pump supplying water to the area. This established that cholera was a waterborne disease.
1863	Jean - Nicolas Demarquay first described the microfilariae which were found in the hydrocele fluid from a Cuban patient.
1872	Timothy Lewis first reported the presence of microfilariae in human blood.
1873	GH Armaeur Hanser in Norway first discovered mycobacterium leprae.
1876	Joseph Bancrofti in Australia recovered the adult worm which was named Filaria bancrofti.
1882	Tubercle bacillus was isolated and described first by Robert Koch.
1884	Diphtheria bacillus was first grown in pure culture by Loeffler.
1885	Louis Pasteur - First developed vaccine for prevention of Rabies.
1897	Ronald Ross reported the presence of pigmented bodies in the gut of mosquitoes that had fed on patients with malaria and later proved the parasitic stage of the life cycle of malaria parasite.
1898	The causative pathogen of Bacillary dysentery was first described by Shiga. Subsequently four species were identified.
19th Century	Plague caused "Black Death" in Europe killing 1/4 to 1/2 of entire population.
1908	Nicolle and Manceaux found the parasite *toxoplasma gondii* in liver and spleen of a North African rodent (*Ctenodactylus* gondi).
1910	Nicolle proved in Algeria in 1910 that typhus is caused by body louse (Louse born typhus). Typhus is derived from Greek word "tyoos" which means fever with stupor or smoke which stands for the "Sanskrit" word "Dhupa".
1933	Lymphocytic choriomenigitis virus was discovered during the study of another epidemic.
1975	Last known case of smallpox in India
1984	WHO in collaboration with UNICEF and many national Governments established the first global control programme against yaws and later against endemic "syphilis" and "pinta".
1993	*Vibrio cholerae* 0139 was first recognized in Indian subcontinent.

Appendix 2

Emerging and Re-emerging Pathogens

Pathogen	Characteristics
Borrelia burgdorferi	It causes Lyme disease. It was first recognized in 1978 in Lyme. Transmission to man occurs through deer ticks, Manifestations include erythema migrans, rash, fever, arthralgia, myalgia, neurological or cardiac symptoms.
Ehrlichia chaffeensis	It causes human monocytic Ehrlichiosis. The pathogen was first recognized in 1987 in Arkansas. The symptoms include fever, rash, arthralgia, and weight loss. Complications include toxic shock-like syndrome and multiorgan failure.
Ehrlichia equi or *Anaplasma Phagocytophilum (Formerly ehrlichia phagocytophilum)*	The pathogen was first recognized in 1992 to 1993. The manifestations are almost the same as in *E. chaffeensis* infection, but rash is less frequent. Case fatality rate may be as high as 10%.
Listeria monocytogenes	A gram-positive bacteria which causes gastrointestinal symptom mostly in immunocompromised or elderly persons.
Vibrio vulnificus	Emergence of the infection was first reported in 1979. Consumption of infected raw oysters results in septicemia, shock and rapid death. Persons with hemochromatosis are particularly vulnerable.
Yersinia enterocolitica	Pigs are the important reservoir. Human transmission is caused by eating infected pork. Usually causes gastroenteritis, sometimes with rectal bleeding and ileal perforation.
Babesia microti	It causes babesisosis and is transmitted to man by tick. Manifestations include fever, mild hepatosplenomegaly, and abdominal pain. Renal failure, adult respiratory distress syndrome and myocardial infarction are the common complications.
Gnathostomosis spinigerum	This nematode has prevalence in South East Asia. Emergence of this infection has been recognized now in Acapulco (Mexico) and South America. Man became infected after ingestion of raw or undercooked fish containing larvae in muscle, especially in ceviche. It causes swelling in man by larva migrans.

Appendix 3

Prevention of Cholera

SUGGESTED MEASURES

1. High standard of personal hygiene is an important safeguard against spread of cholera in the community.
2. Drink safe water preferably from chlorinated sources.
3. Cook all foods thoroughly.
4. Avoid shellfish particularly those from potentially contaminated water.
5. Do not use food and beverages sold by street vendors.
6. Ensure appropriate disposal of human waste.
7. Use acidifying foods like lemons, limes, tomatoes, tamarinds and yoghurt which acidify food and prevent growth of *V. cholerae.*
8. Training of street vendors on sanitation, hygiene and food handling is an important step.
9. Oral vaccines provide short-term protection. However, WHO recommends the use of these vaccines.

Appendix 4

Prevention of Water-borne Infections

1. Safe storage of treated water is essential.
2. Avoid drinking water directly from river, lake or streams.
3. Keep cattle and other animals away from surface water such as river or pond that provides water for drinking.
4. Keep human waste disposal systems like latrines far away from the source of drinking water.
5. Use safe water for brushing teeth.
6. Avoid contact with feces of all animals.
7. Use separate water for washing of utensils and clothes which must not be mixed with drinking water.
8. Avoid swimming in water that is likely to have been contaminated with human or animal waste.
9. Proper flood control, proper treatment, storage and distribution of water should be enforced to ensure safe water supply to the community.
10. Consume only water that has been boiled (not just heated) for one minute or has been treated in some filters.

Appendix 5

Prevention of Food-borne Infections

1. Avoid undercooked meat and poultry.
2. Shell fish should be cooked till shell softens.
3. Avoid raw or undercooked egg or foods containing such eggs.
4. Do not use raw or unpasteurized milk or cheese.
5. Avoid unpasteurized fruit or vegetable juices.
6. Refrigerate left over food promptly.
7. Rinse fresh fruits and vegetables in running tap water to remove dirt.
8. Avoid eating food prepared by nonlicensed street vendors. Hot foods should be used from vendors.
9. Avoid eating food prepared from high-risk animals like game animals, squirrels and rodents.

Appendix 6

Prevention of Rodent-borne Infections

1. Keep the floors and rooms clean from garbage particularly the areas like floor, under almirah, shelf and cots.
2. Discard left over food of pets and empty water bowls.
3. Keep food items in containers with tight cover.
4. Clean grass and bushes in and around the living place.
5. Seal cracks and holes in the floor.
6. Store food for animals in tight covered container.
7. Dispose dead animals properly by burial or burning.
8. Do not sleep near wood piles or garbage areas.
9. Avoid sleeping on bare ground but use mat or cot.
10. Remove junks quickly that are likely to provide shelter to the rodents.

Appendix 7

Prevention of Bite by Mosquitoes

1. Sleep in well-screened areas keeping the unscreened windows closed.
2. Use a mosquito net preferably saturated with an insecticide.
3. Use a spray (permanone) on clothes to repel the mosquitoes.
4. Wear dark colored, long sleeved shirts and long pants.
5. Tightly cover receptacles containing stored water.
6. Dispose the refuse promptly at appropriate place.
7. Eliminate mosquito breeding sites by avoiding water collection in small ditches, old tyres, metal containers, etc.
8. Use household insecticides to keep away insects in living rooms.
9. Avoid sleeping in open spaces in bare body.
10. Use burning coils or candles formulated with mosquito repellant during outdoor lounging.

INDEX

Page numbers followed by *f* refer to figure and *t* refer to table